Paleo Diet Cookbook for Two

2 Books in 1| Paleo Gillian's Meal Plan| 200+ Low Carb Recipes to Improve Your and Your Partner's Body Shape

By Kaylee Gillian

Copyright © 2021 Kaylee Gillian

All rights reserved.

ISBN: 978-1-80321-502-0 (Paperback)

ISBN: 978-1-80321-503-7 (Hardcover)

Table of Contents

Paleo Diet Cookbook for Women

Chapter 1 -   **Introduction** 9

Chapter 2 -   **Breakfast Recipes** 11

1) Tomato and Eggs 12

2) Almond Green Muffins 12

3) Lemony Pancakes 12

4) Coconut Pancakes 13

5) Spiced Waffles 13

6) Vanilla Eggplant Toast 13

7) Coconut Bars 14

8) Chicken and Veggie Rolls 14

9) Turkey and Veggie Frittata 15

10) Coconut Zucchini and Leek Frittata 15

11) Turkey and Beef Patties 15

12) Banana and Nuts Bowls 16

13) Avocado and Pumpkin Sandwich 16

Chapter 3 -   **Soup & Stew Recipes** 17

14) Garlic Tomato and Turkey Soup 18

15) Coconut Tomato Cream Soup 18

16) Rosemary Chicken Soup 18

17) Turmeric Cauliflower Cream 19

18) Herbed Tomato and Beef Soup 19

19) Chili Carrot and Beet Soup 19

20) Celery and Chicken Soup 20

21) Lemon Garlic and Cilantro Soup 20

22) Cilantro Watermelon Soup 20

23) Sweet Potato and Carrot Soup 21

24) Rosemary Mushroom and Beef Stew 21

25) Tomato and Beef Stew 21

26) Lemon Turkey and Zucchini Stew 22

27) Beef and Greens Stew 22

28) Pumpkin and Chicken Stew 22

29) Masala Lamb Stew 23

30) Root Veggie Stew 23

Chapter 4 -   **Side Recipes** 24

31) Balsamic Baked Carrots 25

32) Leeks Mix 25

33) Herbed Mushroom Mix 25

34) Garlic Cauliflower Mix 26

35) Maple and Chili Asparagus 26

36) Garlic Coconut Squash 26

37) Cashew and Chard Mix 27

38) Maple Beets 27

39) Pomegranate and Sprouts Mix 27

40) Cilantro Potatoes 27

Chapter 5 -   **Snack & Appetizer Recipes** 28

41) Chives Cauliflower Bites 29

42) Lemon Cashew Spread 29

43) Avocado Dip 29

44) Lemon Cauliflower Dip 30

45) Tahini Cauliflower Spread 30

46) Lemon Eggplant Hummus 30

47) Cilantro Egg Bites 31

48) Turkey Muffins 31

Paleo Diet Cookbook for Men

Paleo Diet Cookbook for Women

Paleo Gillian's Meal Plan| How to Restore the Ideal Body Shape Without Giving Up Everyday Foods

By Kaylee Gillian

Chapter 1 -   Introduction

Let's talk about the return to the origins of man, what was once the food to eat, not treated, not "bombed" and especially not CULTIVATED!

And what do you do? Do you choose the blue pill and come with me to see what this world was like or do you choose the red pill and stay in the world dominated by the corn empire?

Proteins and Fats

The Paleolithic diet included a higher protein component than is recommended today and differed significantly from the latter. Meat was lean game, poorer and very different in the composition of fats compared to today's meats. Moreover, this food was rich in omega-3 fats, today almost absent in the meat of animals raised on feed (a clear difference from those raised free). Fats are however an essential and important component of the paleolithic diet. Without obviously exaggerating, paleolithic is not synonymous of "excess"...

Carbohydrates

As for the use of carbohydrates, as a source of energy and to restore the acid-base balance of the body, Paleolithic man ate fruits and vegetables, which lead (compared to pasta, rice and bread) to a lower release of insulin, consequently to a lower synthesis of fats. Carbohydrates with A.I.G. (high glycemic index), in fact, those derived from cereals, are responsible for the rapid rise in the concentration of glucose in the blood (blood sugar), an event that triggers the "perverse mechanism of insulin".

So, to recap, the tips for a good paleolithic diet are:

Have many small meals and not a few large ones; this also reduces hormonal (insulin) stimulation compared to that caused by larger, more concentrated meals.

Eat red or white meat (even if today's meat is treated compared to millions of years ago and loses many nutritional values compared to the paleolithic one; it is not a coincidence that farm animals are given feed with cereals inside, when they were free, however, they ate what nature had imposed) and carbohydrates taken from fruits and vegetables, avoiding pasta, bread, cookies, rusks, rice and all derivatives of cereals

Dissociate foods correctly, that is avoid mixing different proteins, in this way each food will be better digested and absorbed by the body.

Do physical activity: Paleolithic man went to hunt for food, he did not sit on a sofa watching TV, and made a fight to kill the animal; now instead we go to the supermarket and everything is already ready, so it is very important to do some sport.

With this diet, also associated with a zone diet, I was able to "bring back to the roots" many people in a short time, devastated by dietary regimes that unfortunately today's society imposes on us. Happy re-entry into today's civilization or happy beginning of a new era...paleo!

Chapter 2 - Breakfast Recipes

1) Tomato and Eggs

Preparation Time: 10 minutes   **Cooking Time: 30 minutes**   **Servings:2**

Ingredients:

- 2 eggs
- 2 tomatoes

- A pinch of salt and black pepper
- 1 teaspoon parsley, finely chopped

Directions:

⇒ Cut tomatoes tops, scoop flesh, arrange them on a lined baking sheet, and crack an egg in each tomato.

⇒ Season with salt and pepper.

⇒ Place the baking sheet in the oven at 350 degrees F and bake for 30 minutes.

⇒ Take tomatoes out of the oven, divide between plates, sprinkle parsley at the end and serve.

Nutrition: calories 85, fat 4,6, fiber 1,5, carbs 5,2, protein 6,7, fat 4,6, sugar 3,6

2) Almond Green Muffins

Preparation Time: 10 minutes   **Cooking Time: 30 minutes**   **Servings:4**

Ingredients:

- 1 cup kale, chopped
- ¼ cup chives, finely chopped
- ½ cup almond milk

- 6 eggs
- Black pepper to taste
- Cooking spray

Directions:

⇒ In a bowl, mix the eggs with chives, kale, the milk and black pepper and whisk well.

⇒ Divide this into 8 muffin cups after you've greased them with cooking spray.

⇒ Place the muffin cups in a preheated oven at 350 degrees F and bake for 30 minutes.

⇒ Take muffins out of the oven, leave them to cool down, transfer them to plates and serve warm for breakfast

Nutrition: calories 174, fat 13,9, fiber 1, carbs 4,1, protein 9,6, sugar 1,6

3) Lemony Pancakes

Preparation Time: 10 minutes   **Cooking Time: 10 minutes**   **Servings:2**

Ingredients:

- 4 eggs
- 2 bananas, peeled and chopped
- ¼ teaspoon baking soda

- 2 tablespoons lemon juice
- Cooking spray

Directions:

⇒ In a blender, mix eggs with the bananas, baking soda, and lemon juice, and pulse well.

⇒ Heat a pan greased with cooking spray over a medium-high heat, add half of the batter, spread into the pan, cook for 1 minute on each side and transfer to a plate.

⇒ Repeat this with the rest of the batter and serve for breakfast.

Nutrition: calories 237, fat 9,5, fiber 3,1, carbs 28, sugar 15,4, protein 12,5

4) Coconut Pancakes

Preparation Time: 10 minutes   **Cooking Time: 10 minutes**   **Servings:2**

Ingredients:

- 3 eggs
- ¼ cup coconut flour
- ¼ cup coconut water
- 1 teaspoon coconut oil
- ½ plantain, peeled and chopped

- ¼ teaspoon baking soda
- ¼ teaspoon chai spice
- 1 tablespoon shaved coconut, toasted for serving
- 1 tablespoon coconut milk for serving

Directions:

⇒ In a food processor, mix eggs with coconut water and flour, plantain, baking soda and chai spice and blend well.

⇒ Heat up a pan with the oil over a medium heat, add ¼ cup pancake batter, spread evenly, cook until it becomes golden, flip pancake and cook for 1 more minute and transfer to a plate.

⇒ Repeat this with the rest of the batter, divide all the pancakes between plates and serve with the coconut and coconut milk.

Nutrition: calories 253, fat 12,9, fiber 6,5, carbs 24,5, protein 11,3 sugar 9,4

5) Spiced Waffles

Preparation Time: 10 minutes   **Cooking Time: 10 minutes**   **Servings:4**

Ingredients:

- 2 sweet potatoes, peeled and finely grated
- 2 tablespoons coconut oil, melted
- 3 eggs

- 1 teaspoon cinnamon powder
- ½ teaspoon nutmeg, ground

Directions:

⇒ In a bowl, mix the eggs with sweet potatoes, coconut oil, cinnamon and nutmeg and whisk well.

⇒ Cook waffles in your waffle iron, divide between plates and serve.

Nutrition: calories 225, fat 10,4, fiber 4,2, carbs 28,3, sugar 0,8, protein 5,7

6) Vanilla Eggplant Toast

Preparation Time: 5 minutes   **Cooking Time: 6 minutes**   **Servings:2**

Ingredients:

- 1 eggplant, peeled and sliced
- 1 teaspoon vanilla extract
- 2 eggs

- 1 teaspoon stevia
- 1 teaspoon coconut oil, melted

Directions:

⇒ In a bowl, mix the eggs with vanilla, stevia to taste, and cinnamon and whisk well.

⇒ Heat up a pan with the coconut oil over medium-high heat.

⇒ Dip eggplant slices in eggs mix, add to the pan, cook them for 3 minutes on each side, divide between plates and serve for breakfast.

Nutrition: calories 146, fat 7,1, fiber 8,1, carbs 14,1, protein 7,8

7)   Coconut Bars

Preparation Time: 10 minutes   **Cooking Time: 15 minutes**   **Servings:6**

Ingredients:

- 5 ounces dates, soaked in hot water
- Juice of 1 orange
- Grated rind of ½ orange
- 1 cup desiccated coconut

- ½ cup silvered almonds
- ½ cup pumpkin seeds
- ½ cup sesame seeds

Directions:

⇒ In a bowl, mix the almonds with orange rind, orange juice, coconut, pumpkin and sesame seeds and stir well.

⇒ Drain dates, add them to a food processor, blend well, add this over the orange mixture and stir everything.

⇒ Spread this on a lined baking sheet, place in the oven at 350 degrees F and bake for 15 minutes, stirring every 4 minutes.

⇒ Take granola out of the oven, leave aside to cool down, cut into bars and serve for breakfast.

Nutrition: calories 427, fat 32,3, fiber 8,8, carbs 32,1, protein 10,1

8)   Chicken and Veggie Rolls

Preparation Time: 10 minutes   **Cooking Time: 10 minutes**   **Servings:4**

Ingredients:

- 1 small yellow onion, chopped
- 4 eggs, egg yolks and whites separated
- 0,5 oz green chilies, chopped
- 2 tomatoes, chopped
- 1 red bell pepper, cut into thin strips

- ¼ cup cilantro, chopped
- ½ cup rotisserie chicken, already cooked and shredded, paleo friendly
- Black pepper to taste
- 2 tablespoons olive oil
- 1 avocado, pitted, peeled and chopped

Directions:

⇒ Put egg whites in a bowl, add black pepper, whisk well and leave them to one side.

⇒ Heat up a pan with half of the oil over medium-high heat, add half of the egg whites, spread evenly, cover pan, cook for 2 minutes and then slide on a plate.

⇒ Repeat this with the rest of the egg whites and leave the two "egg tortillas" aside.

⇒ Heat up the same pan with the rest of the oil over medium-high heat, add onions, stir and cook for 2 minutes.

⇒ Add red bell pepper, green chilies, tomato, meat and cilantro and stir.

⇒ Add egg yolks to the pan and scramble the whole mix for 4-5 minutes

⇒ Add avocado, stir, take off the heat, spread evenly on the two "tortillas", roll them, divide between plates and serve for breakfast.

Nutrition: calories 274, fat 4,9, fiber 4,9, carbs 11,4, protein 11,9

9) Turkey and Veggie Frittata

Preparation Time: 10 minutes   **Cooking Time: 30 minutes**   **Servings:4**

Ingredients:

- ½ pound turkey meat, cooked, minced
- 2 tablespoons olive oil
- 1 cup white mushrooms, sliced
- 1 cup spinach leaves, chopped
- 10 eggs, whisked
- 1 yellow onion, finely chopped
- Black pepper to taste

Directions:

⇒ Heat up a pan with the oil over medium-high heat, add the onion, stir and brown for 3 minutes

⇒ Add the turkey meat, stir and cook for 10 minutes more.

⇒ Add the spinach and mushrooms and cook for 4 minutes.

⇒ Take the pan off the heat, add the eggs and some black pepper, spread evenly, place the frittata in the oven at 350 degrees F, bake for 20 minutes, divide between plates and serve for breakfast.

Nutrition: calories 330, fat 20,9, fiber 1, carbs 4,3, protein 31,5

10) Coconut Zucchini and Leek Frittata

Preparation Time: 10 minutes   **Cooking Time: 40 minutes**   **Servings:4**

Ingredients:

- 10 eggs, whisked
- Black pepper to taste
- ¼ cup coconut cream
- 1 yellow onion, finely chopped
- 1 leek, thinly sliced
- 2 scallions, thinly sliced
- 2 zucchinis, cubed
- 8 zucchini flowers
- 2 tablespoons avocado oil

Directions:

⇒ In a bowl, mix the eggs with coconut cream and black pepper then whisk.

⇒ Heat up a pan with the oil over a medium heat, add the leek and onions, stir and sauté for 5 minutes.

⇒ Add the zucchini, stir and cook for 10 more minutes.

⇒ Add the eggs mix, spread, reduce heat to low, and cook for 5 minutes.

⇒ Sprinkle scallions and arrange the zucchini flowers on top of the frittata, place in the oven at 350 degrees F and bake for 20 minutes.

⇒ Slice the frittata, divide between plates and serve for breakfast.

Nutrition: calories 384, fat 24,8, fiber 4,9, carbs 23,7, protein 18,2

11) Turkey and Beef Patties

Preparation Time: 10 minutes   **Cooking Time: 20 minutes**   **Servings:4**

Ingredients:

- 5 eggs
- 1 pound ground beef meat
- ½ cup turkey meat, minced
- 4 small shallots
- 3 sun-dried tomatoes, chopped
- 2 teaspoons basil leaves, chopped
- 1 teaspoon garlic, minced
- A drizzle of olive oil
- Black pepper to taste

Directions:

⇒ In a bowl, combine the meat with 1 egg, tomatoes, basil, black pepper and garlic, stir and shape 4 burgers.

⇒ Heat up a pan over medium-high heat, add the burgers, cook them 5 minutes on each side and transfer them to a plate.

⇒ Heat up the same pan over medium-high heat, place the turkey patties, cook for 20 minutes and transfer it to a plate as well.

⇒ Heat up the pan again, add the chopped shallots and extra olive oil, cook for 4 minutes, drain excess oil and add next to the turkey patties.

⇒ Fry the remaining eggs in a pan with a drizzle of oil over a medium-high heat and place them on top of the burgers.

⇒ Top with the turkey patties and shallots and serve for breakfast.

Nutrition: calories 406, fat 18,1, carbs 14,8, fiber 1,1, protein 45,5

12) Banana and Nuts Bowls

Preparation Time: 5 minutes   **Cooking Time: 5 minutes**   **Servings:2**

Ingredients:

- 2 tablespoons coconut butter
- ½ cup walnuts, soaked for 2 hours and drained
- ¾ cup hot water

- 1 banana, peeled and chopped
- ½ teaspoon cinnamon powder
- 2 teaspoons coconut sugar

Directions:

⇒ Put all the ingredients in a blender, and pulse well.

⇒ Transfer this to a pan, heat up over medium heat until it thickens, divide into bowls and serve for breakfast.

Nutrition: calories 447, fat 36,6, fiber 8,7, carbs 27,8, protein 10,2

13) Avocado and Pumpkin Sandwich

Preparation Time: 10 minutes   **Cooking Time: 10 minutes**   **Servings:2**

Ingredients:

- 4 ounces pumpkin flesh, peeled
- 4 slices paleo coconut bread
- 1 avocado, pitted and peeled

- 1 carrot, grated
- 2 lettuce leaves

Directions:

⇒ Spread the pumpkin flesh in a tray, bake at 350 degrees F for 10 minutes, transfer to a bowl and mash it with a fork.

⇒ Put the avocado in separate bowl and mash it with a fork.

⇒ Spread avocado on 2 paleo bread slices, also divide the grated carrot, mashed pumpkin and the lettuce leaves on each and top them with the other 2 bread slices and serve for breakfast.

Nutrition: calories 310, fat 21,7, fiber 20,1, carbs 26,6, protein 12,6

Chapter 3 -   Soup & Stew Recipes

14) Garlic Tomato and Turkey Soup

Preparation Time: 15 minutes   **Cooking Time: 40 minutes**   **Servings:6**

Ingredients:

- 1 yellow onion, chopped
- 1 tablespoon avocado oil
- 3 thyme springs, chopped
- 3 garlic cloves, finely minced
- 25 oz fresh tomatoes, peeled, chopped
- 6 ounces tomato paste
- ¼ cup water
- 1 pound turkey meat, ground, fried
- 14 ounces beef stock
- 6 mushrooms, chopped
- 1 small red bell pepper, chopped
- ½ cup black olives, chopped

Directions:

⇒ Heat a saucepan with the oil over medium-high heat, add half of the onion, garlic and thyme. Stir and cook for 5 minutes.

⇒ Add tomatoes, tomato paste and the water, stir, bring to a boil, reduce heat to medium-low and simmer for 20 minutes.

⇒ Pour this mixture into a blender and pulse well.

⇒ Heat up a saucepan over medium-high heat, add the turkey, stir and cook for 4 minutes, breaking it into small pieces with a fork.

⇒ Add the rest of the onion, mushrooms and the bell pepper, stir and cook for 5 minutes.

⇒ Add blended soup and beef stock, stir and cook for 5 more minutes.

⇒ Ladle the soup into bowls, top with the olives and serve.

Nutrition: calories 218, fat 6, fiber 4,6, carbs 16,3, protein 18,3

15) Coconut Tomato Cream Soup

Preparation Time: 10 minutes   **Cooking Time: 35 minutes**   **Servings:4**

Ingredients:

- 56 oz fresh tomatoes, peeled, crushed
- 2 cups tomato juice
- 2 cups chicken stock
- ¼ pound coconut butter, melted
- 14 basil leaves, torn
- 1 cup coconut milk
- Salt and black pepper to the taste

Directions:

⇒ Put tomatoes, tomato juice and stock in a saucepan, heat up over medium-high heat, bring to a boil, reduce heat, stir and simmer for 30 minutes.

⇒ Pour this into a blender, add basil, pulse very well and return to saucepan.

⇒ Heat up the soup again, add the butter, salt, pepper and coconut milk, stir, cook over low heat for 4 minutes more, divide into bowls and serve.

Nutrition: calories 421, fat 33,5, fiber 11,6, carbs 31,3, protein 8,2

16) Rosemary Chicken Soup

Preparation Time: 15 minutes   **Cooking Time: 60 minutes**   **Servings:4**

Ingredients:

- 2 teaspoons coconut oil, melted
- 3 carrots, chopped
- 1 yellow onion, chopped
- 1 zucchini, chopped
- 15 ounces mushrooms, chopped
- 4 cups chicken meat, already cooked and shredded
- 2 teaspoons rosemary, dried
- 1 teaspoon thyme, dried
- 1 tablespoon apple cider vinegar
- 1 teaspoon cumin, ground
- 2 and ½ cups chicken stock
- A pinch of sea salt and black pepper

Directions:

⇒ Heat up a saucepan with the oil over medium heat, add carrots and onion, stir and cook for 5 minutes.

⇒ Add zucchini, and mushrooms, stir and cook for 10 more minutes.

⇒ Add the chicken meat, rosemary, thyme, vinegar, cumin and the stock, stir, bring to a boil, reduce heat to medium-low and simmer for 40 minutes.

⇒ Add salt and pepper to the taste, stir again, ladle into bowls and serve.

Nutrition: calories 459, fat 16,9, carbs 23,6, protein 52,8, fiber 3,7

17) Turmeric Cauliflower Cream

Preparation Time: 10 minutes   **Cooking Time: 60 minutes**   **Servings:6**

Ingredients:

- 1 yellow onion, chopped
- 2 tablespoons extra virgin olive oil
- 2 pounds cauliflower florets
- A pinch of sea salt and black pepper
- ½ teaspoon turmeric powder
- 2 garlic cloves, minced
- 5 cups veggie stock

Directions:

⇒ Heat up a saucepan with the oil over medium heat, add the onion and garlic, stir and sauté for 10 minutes.

⇒ Add cauliflower, salt and pepper, stir and cook for 12 more minutes.

⇒ Add the stock, stir, bring to a boil, reduce heat to medium and simmer for 25 minutes.

⇒ Transfer to a blender, add the turmeric powder, pulse well, ladle into bowls and serve.

Nutrition: calories 100, fat 6,8, carbs 12,4, fiber 4,3, protein 3,3

18) Herbed Tomato and Beef Soup

Preparation Time: 10 minutes   **Cooking Time: 1 hour**   **Servings:6**

Ingredients:

- 2 pounds organic beef, ground
- 4 cups beef stock
- 25 oz fresh tomatoes, peeled, chopped
- 1 green bell pepper, chopped
- 3 zucchinis, chopped
- 1 cup celery, chopped
- 1 teaspoon Italian seasoning
- ½ yellow onion, chopped
- ½ teaspoon oregano, dried
- ½ teaspoon basil, dried
- ¼ teaspoon garlic powder
- A pinch of sea salt and black pepper

Directions:

⇒ Heat up a saucepan over medium heat, add the beef, stir, cook for 5 minutes and drain excess grease

⇒ Add all the other ingredients, reduce heat to medium-low and simmer for 1 hour.

⇒ Ladle the soup into bowls and serve right away.

Nutrition: calories 345, fat 10,5, fiber 3,3, carbs 11,1, protein 50,4

19) Chili Carrot and Beet Soup

Preparation Time: 10 minutes   **Cooking Time: 1 hour and 30 minutes**   **Servings:8**

Ingredients:

- 1 sweet onion, chopped
- 2 tablespoons ghee, melted
- 5 carrots, chopped
- 3 parsnips, chopped
- 3 beets, chopped
- 3 small shallots, chopped, cooked and crumbled
- 1-quart chicken stock
- A pinch of sea salt and black pepper
- 2 quarts water
- ½ teaspoon chili flakes
- 1 tablespoons rosemary, chopped

Directions:

⇒ Heat up a Dutch oven with the ghee over medium-high heat, add the onion, stir and cook for 5 minutes.

⇒ Add all the other ingredients, stir, bring to a boil, reduce heat to medium-low and simmer for 1 hour and 30 minutes.

⇒ Ladle the soup into bowls and serve hot.

Nutrition: calories 139, fat 3,9, fiber 6,2, carbs 25,4, protein 2,6

20) Celery and Chicken Soup

Preparation Time: 15 minutes   **Cooking Time: 30 minutes**   **Servings:6**

Ingredients:

- 2 celery stalks, chopped
- ½ cup coconut oil, melted
- 2 carrots, chopped
- ½ cup arrowroot powder
- 6 cups chicken stock
- 1 teaspoon parsley, dried
- ½ cup water

- 1 bay leaf
- A pinch of sea salt and black pepper
- ½ teaspoon thyme, dried
- 1 and ½ cups coconut milk
- 3 cups organic chicken meat, already cooked and cubed

Directions:

⇒ Heat up a large saucepan with the oil over medium-high heat, add carrots and celery, stir and cook for 10 minutes.

⇒ Add stock, stir and bring to a boil.

⇒ In a bowl, mix arrowroot with ½ cup water, whisk well and add to the pot.

⇒ Also add parsley, sea salt, pepper, bay leaf and thyme, stir and simmer over medium heat for 15 minutes.

⇒ Add the meat and coconut milk, stir, cook 1 more minute, ladle into bowls and serve.

Nutrition: calories 793, fat 71,7, fiber 5,1, carbs 19,6, protein 25,8

21) Lemon Garlic and Cilantro Soup

Preparation Time: 10 minutes   **Cooking Time: 10 minutes**   **Servings:4**

Ingredients:

- 6 cups shellfish stock
- 1 tablespoons garlic, minced
- 1 tablespoon coconut oil, melted
- 2 eggs

- ½ cup lemon juice
- A pinch of sea salt and black pepper
- 1 tablespoon arrowroot powder
- 1 tablespoon cilantro, chopped

Directions:

⇒ Heat up a saucepan with the oil over medium-high heat, add the garlic, stir and cook for 2 minutes.

⇒ Add the stock, stir and bring to a simmer.

⇒ In a bowl, mix eggs with salt, pepper, lemon juice and arrowroot, whisk very well, pour into the pot, stir, cook for 4 minutes more, ladle into bowls and serve with chopped cilantro on top.

Nutrition: calories 64, fat 4,7, carbs 5, fiber 0,2, protein 1,8

22) Cilantro Watermelon Soup

Preparation Time: 10 minutes   **Cooking Time:**   **Servings:3**

Ingredients:

- 1 avocado, pitted and chopped
- 1 cucumber, chopped
- 2 bunches spinach
- 1 and ½ cups watermelon, chopped

- 1 bunch cilantro, roughly chopped
- Juice of 2 lemons
- ½ cup coconut aminos
- ½ cup lime juice

Directions:

⇒ In your blender, combine all the ingredients, pulse them well, divide into bowls and serve.

Nutrition: calories 288, fat 14,2, carbs 42,9, fiber 11,8, protein 9,5

23) Sweet Potato and Carrot Soup

Preparation Time: 10 minutes   **Cooking Time: 45 minutes**   **Servings:4**

Ingredients:

- 2 sweet potatoes, peeled and chopped
- 2 yellow onions, cut into wedges
- 2 pounds carrots, diced
- 4 tablespoons coconut oil, melted

- 1 head garlic, cloves peeled
- A pinch of sea salt and black pepper
- 2 cups chicken stock
- 3 tablespoons maple syrup

Directions:

⇒ Put onions, carrots, sweet potatoes and garlic in a baking dish, add the oil, salt and pepper, toss to coat, place in the oven at 425 degrees F and bake for 35 minutes.

⇒ Transfer the veggies to a large saucepan, add chicken stock, heat everything over medium-high heat, reduce to medium-low and cook for 10 minutes.

⇒ Transfer soup to a blender, pulse well, divide into soup bowls and serve.

Nutrition: calories 371, fat 14,1, carbs 60,3, fiber 9,9, protein 4,3

24) Rosemary Mushroom and Beef Stew

Preparation Time: 10 minutes   **Cooking Time: 2 hours**   **Servings:4**

Ingredients:

- 2 pounds beef stew meat, cubed
- 1 red chili, seeded and chopped
- 1 brown onion, chopped
- 1 teaspoon ghee, melted
- 2 tablespoons extra virgin olive oil
- A pinch of sea salt and black pepper
- 2/3 teaspoon nutmeg, ground
- 1 garlic clove, minced

- ½ cup white mushrooms, sliced
- 1 teaspoon rosemary, dried
- ¼ teaspoon fennel seeds
- 2 celery stick, chopped
- 2 carrots, thinly sliced
- 1-quart beef stock
- 2 tablespoons almond flour
- 1 sweet potato, chopped

Directions:

⇒ Heat up a large saucepan with the ghee and the olive oil over medium-high heat, add onion, chili, salt and pepper, stir and cook for 2-3 minutes.

⇒ Add the meat, stir and brown it for 5 minutes.

⇒ Add the mushrooms, garlic, stock, fennel, rosemary and the nutmeg, stir, bring to a boil, cover, reduce heat to low and cook for 1 hour and 10 minutes.

⇒ Add celery, carrots, and the potato, stir, cover and cook for 30 minutes.

⇒ In a bowl, mix the flour with a cup of liquid from the stew, stir well, pour over the stew, cook for 15 more minutes, divide into bowls and serve.

Nutrition: calories 574, fat 23,6, carbs 13,8, fiber 3,3, protein 73,5

25) Tomato and Beef Stew

Preparation Time: 10 minutes   **Cooking Time: 8 hours**   **Servings:6**

Ingredients:

- 2 pounds beef stew meat, cubed
- 3 cups beef stock
- 7 garlic cloves, minced
- A pinch of sea salt and black pepper
- 4 carrots, chopped

- 1 cup coconut flour
- 2 yellow onions, chopped
- ½ green cabbage head, chopped
- 25 ounces tomatoes, peeled, chopped

Directions:

⇒ In a slow cooker, combine all the ingredients, toss, cover and cook on Low for 8 hours.

⇒ Divide into bowls and serve.

Nutrition: calories 412, fat 11,3, carbs 25, fiber 9,8, protein 21,7

26) Lemon Turkey and Zucchini Stew

Preparation Time: 10 minutes   **Cooking Time: 30 minutes**   **Servings:3**

Ingredients:

- 1 yellow onion, chopped
- 1 tablespoon coconut oil, melted
- 15 ounces turkey meat, cooked, thinly sliced
- 1 red bell pepper, chopped
- 1 carrot, thinly sliced
- 1 celery stick, chopped
- 1 tomato, chopped

- 2 garlic cloves, minced
- 2 cups chicken stock
- 1 tablespoon lemon juice
- Black pepper to the taste
- 1 zucchini, chopped
- A handful parsley leaves, chopped

Directions:

⇒ Heat up a pan with the oil over medium-high heat, add turkey, onion, celery and carrot, stir and cook for 3 minutes.

⇒ Add red bell pepper, tomatoes and garlic, stir and cook 1 minute.

⇒ Add lemon juice, stock and pepper, stir, bring to a boil, cover pan, reduce heat to medium and cook for 10 minutes.

⇒ Add zucchini, stir, cook for 12 more minutes, divide into bowls, sprinkle the parsley on top and serve.

Nutrition: calories 345, fat 12,4, fiber 3,3, carbs 13,5, protein 44,3

27) Beef and Greens Stew

Preparation Time: 10 minutes   **Cooking Time: 5 hours**   **Servings:4**

Ingredients:

- 6 plantains, skinless and cubed
- 2 pounds beef meat, cubed
- 3 cups collard greens, chopped
- A pinch of sea salt and black pepper
- 3 cups water

- ½ cup sweet paprika
- 3 tablespoons allspice
- ¼ cup garlic powder
- 1 teaspoon chili powder
- 1 teaspoon cayenne pepper

Directions:

⇒ In a slow cooker, mix all the ingredients, toss, cover and cook on High for 5 hours.

⇒ Divide into bowls and serve.

Nutrition: calories 827, fat 19,6, fiber 14,2, carbs 104,5, protein 19,9

28) Pumpkin and Chicken Stew

Preparation Time: 15 minutes   **Cooking Time: 8 hours**   **Servings:6**

Ingredients:

- 5 garlic cloves, minced
- 2 celery stalks, chopped
- 2 yellow onions, chopped
- 2 carrots, chopped
- 30 ounces homemade pumpkin puree
- 2 quarts chicken stock

- 2 cups chicken breast, skinless, boneless and cubed
- ¼ cup coconut flour
- Black pepper to taste
- ½ pound baby spinach
- ¼ teaspoon cayenne pepper

Directions:

⇒ In a slow cooker, combine all the ingredients except the spinach, cover and cook on Low for 7 hours and 50 minutes.

⇒ Add the spinach, cook on Low for 10 more minutes, divide into bowls and serve.

Nutrition: calories 222, fat 3,6, fiber 10,8, carbs 30, protein 18,6

29) Masala Lamb Stew

Preparation Time: 15 minutes   **Cooking Time: 1 hour and 50 minutes**   **Servings:4**

Ingredients:

- 1 and ½ pounds lamb meat, cubed
- 1 tablespoon coconut oil, melted
- ½ red chili, seedless and chopped
- 1 brown onion, chopped
- 3 garlic cloves, minced
- 2 celery sticks, chopped
- 2 and ½ teaspoons garam masala powder
- 1 teaspoon fennel seeds

- A pinch of sea salt and black pepper
- 1 and ¼ teaspoons turmeric powder
- 1 and ½ teaspoons ghee, melted
- 14 ounces coconut milk
- 1 cup water
- 1 tablespoon lemon juice
- 2 carrots, chopped
- A handful parsley leaves, finely chopped

Directions:

⇒ Heat up a pan with the oil over medium-high heat, add the lamb, stir and brown for 4 minutes.

⇒ Add celery, chili and onion, stir and cook 1 minute more.

⇒ Reduce heat to medium, add garam masala, garlic, ghee, fennel, and turmeric, stir and cook 1 minute.

⇒ Add salt, pepper, tomato paste, coconut milk and water, stir, bring to a boil, reduce heat to low, cover and cook for 1 hour.

⇒ Add carrots and cook for 40 minutes more, stirring occasionally.

⇒ Add lemon juice and parsley, stir, transfer to bowls and serve.

Nutrition: calories 829, fat 54, fiber 9,5, carbs 38,7, protein 45,1

30) Root Veggie Stew

Preparation Time: 10 minutes   **Cooking Time: 1 hour and 10 minutes**   **Servings:6**

Ingredients:

- 4 pounds mixed root vegetables (parsnips, carrots, rutabagas, beets, celery root, turnips), chopped
- 6 tablespoons extra virgin olive oil
- 1 garlic head, cloves separated and peeled
- ½ cup yellow onion, chopped

- Black pepper to taste
- 25 ounces fresh tomatoes, peeled, chopped
- 1 tablespoon tomato paste
- 2 cups kale leaves, torn
- 1 teaspoon oregano, dried

Directions:

⇒ In a baking dish, mix all root vegetables with black pepper, half of the oil and garlic, toss to coat, and bake at 450 degrees F for 45 minutes.

⇒ Heat up a pot with the rest of the oil over medium-high heat, add onions and sauté for 2-3 minutes

⇒ Add tomato paste, tomatoes, salt, pepper and the oregano, stir, bring to a simmer, reduce heat to low and cook for 10 minutes.

⇒ Add baked veggies and kale, toss, cook for 5 more minutes, divide into bowls and serve.

Nutrition: calories 293, fat 19,2, fiber 9,8, carbs 32,7, protein 2,2

Chapter 4 -   Side Recipes

31) Balsamic Baked Carrots

Preparation Time: 10 minutes   **Cooking Time: 30 minutes**   **Servings:4**

Ingredients:

- 1 and ½ pounds young carrots (yellow, purple and red ones)
- 2 tablespoons balsamic vinegar
- 2 garlic cloves, finely minced
- 2 tablespoons coconut oil, melted
- A pinch of sea salt and black pepper
- 1 tablespoon coconut sugar
- 1 tablespoon parsley, chopped

Directions:

⇒ In a bowl, combine all the ingredients except the parsley, toss, transfer everything to a baking dish, and bake at 400 degrees F for 30 minutes.

⇒ Divide the carrots between plates, sprinkle the parsley on top and serve as a side dish.

Nutrition: calories 123, fat 7, fiber 4;4, carbs 15, protein 1,1

32) Leeks Mix

Preparation Time: 10 minutes   **Cooking Time: 10 minutes**   **Servings:4**

Ingredients:

- 2 zucchinis, sliced
- 2 leeks, sliced lengthwise
- ¼ cup extra virgin olive oil
- 1/3 cup walnuts, toasted and chopped
- ¼ cup cilantro, chopped
- ¼ cup parsley, chopped
- A pinch of sea salt and black pepper
- Juice of 1 lemon
- 2 garlic cloves, minced

Directions:

⇒ Season leeks and zucchinis with salt and pepper, arrange them on your pre-heated grill over medium-high heat and cook them for 8 minutes, flipping them from time to time.

⇒ Transfer veggies to a bowl, add walnuts, parsley, oil, cilantro, garlic and lemon juice, toss to coat and serve as a side dish.

Nutrition: calories 222, fat 19,2, fiber 2,8, carbs 12,4, protein 4,7

33) Herbed Mushroom Mix

Preparation Time: 10 minutes   **Cooking Time: 4 hours**   **Servings:4**

Ingredients:

- 4 garlic cloves, finely minced
- ¼ teaspoon thyme, dried
- ½ teaspoon basil, dried
- ½ teaspoon oregano, dried
- 24 ounces cremini mushrooms
- 2 tablespoons parsley, chopped
- ¼ cup coconut milk
- 1 cup veggie stock
- 2 tablespoons ghee, melted
- A pinch of sea salt and black pepper

Directions:

⇒ In a slow cooker, combine all the ingredients, cover and cook on Low for 4 hours.

⇒ Divide between plates and serve as a side dish.

Nutrition: calories 145, fat 10,7, fiber 1,6, carbs 9,6, protein 4,9

34) Garlic Cauliflower Mix

Preparation Time: 10 minutes   **Cooking Time: 20 minutes**   **Servings:4**

Ingredients:

- 2 garlic cloves, finely chopped
- 6 cups cauliflower florets
- 2 green onions, thinly sliced

- A pinch of sea salt and black pepper
- 3 tablespoons ghee

Directions:

⇒ Put water in a large saucepan, place on stove over medium-high heat, bring to a boil, add the cauliflower, cook for 20 minutes and drain the water.

⇒ Add salt, pepper and the ghee and mash everything using a hand mixer.

⇒ Divide between plates, sprinkle chopped green onions on top and serve as a side dish.

Nutrition: calories 126, fat 9,7, fiber 4, carbs 9, protein 3,2

35) Maple and Chili Asparagus

Preparation Time: 10 minutes   **Cooking Time: 10 minutes**   **Servings:4**

Ingredients:

- 1 and ½ pounds asparagus, trimmed
- A pinch of sea salt and black pepper
- 2 garlic cloves, minced
- 1 shallot, finely chopped
- ½ teaspoon red chili flakes

- 2 teaspoons mustard
- 1 teaspoon maple syrup
- 2 tablespoons ghee, melted
- 2 teaspoons balsamic vinegar

Directions:

⇒ In a bowl, mix vinegar with mustard, maple syrup, salt and pepper and whisk.

⇒ Heat up a pan with the ghee over medium-high heat, add garlic, shallots and pepper flakes, stir and cook for 2 minutes.

⇒ Add asparagus, stir and cook for 5 minutes.

⇒ Add the vinegar, toss to coat, cook for 3 minutes more, divide between plates and serve as a side dish.

Nutrition: calories 110, fat 7,1, fiber 3,8, carbs 10, protein 4,4

36) Garlic Coconut Squash

Preparation Time: 10 minutes   **Cooking Time: 40 minutes**   **Servings:4**

Ingredients:

- 2 tablespoons coconut oil, melted
- 1 butternut squash, peeled and chopped
- 3 garlic cloves, finely minced

- 1 tablespoon thyme, chopped
- A pinch of sea salt and black pepper

Directions:

⇒ Heat up a pan with the oil over medium-high heat, add garlic, squash, and thyme, stir and cook for 10 minutes.

⇒ Reduce the heat to medium low, and cook for 10 more minutes, stirring from time to time.

⇒ Add salt and pepper, stir again, divide between plates and serve as a side dish.

Nutrition: calories 80, fat 6,9, fiber 1, carbs 5,3, protein 0,6

37) Cashew and Chard Mix

Preparation Time: 10 minutes   **Cooking Time: 10 minutes**   **Servings:2**

Ingredients:

- ½ cup cashews, chopped
- 1 bunch chard, cut into thin strips
- A pinch of sea salt and black pepper
- 1 tablespoon coconut oil, melted

Directions:

⇒ Heat up a pan with the oil over medium heat, add the chard and cashews, stir and cook for 10 minutes.

⇒ Add salt and pepper stir, cook for 1 minute more, take off heat, divide between plates and serve as a side dish.

Nutrition: calories 260, fat 22,7, fiber 1,4, carbs 12,1, protein 5,7

38) Maple Beets

Preparation Time: 10 minutes   **Cooking Time: 50 minutes**   **Servings:4**

Ingredients:

- 2 tablespoons extra virgin olive oil
- 6 beets, cut into quarters and sliced
- A pinch of sea salt and black pepper
- ½ cup balsamic vinegar
- 1 teaspoon orange zest, grated
- 2 teaspoons maple syrup

Directions:

⇒ Arrange beets on a lined baking sheet, add salt, pepper and the olive oil, toss, and bake in the oven at 325 degrees F for 45 minutes.

⇒ Heat up a pan over medium heat, add the vinegar and maple syrup, whisk and cook for 2 minutes.

⇒ Divide the beets between plates, drizzle the vinegar mix all over, sprinkle the orange zest and serve right away as a side dish.

Nutrition: calories 141, fat 7,3, fiber 3,1, carbs 17,6, protein 2,5

39) Pomegranate and Sprouts Mix

Preparation Time: 10 minutes   **Cooking Time: 30 minutes**   **Servings:6**

Ingredients:

- 1 and ½ pounds Brussels sprouts, halved
- A pinch of sea salt and black pepper
- 1 teaspoon garlic powder
- 2/3 cups pecans, chopped
- 1 cup pomegranate seeds
- 2 tablespoons extra virgin olive oil

Directions:

⇒ In a baking dish, combine all the ingredients except the pomegranate seeds, toss and bake at 400 degrees F for 30 minutes.

⇒ Divide between plates, top with pomegranate seeds and serve as a side dish.

Nutrition: calories 184, fat 13,4, fiber 5,3, carbs 15,3, protein 5

40) Cilantro Potatoes

Preparation Time: 10 minutes   **Cooking Time: 45 minutes**   **Servings:4**

Ingredients:

- 3 sweet potatoes, pricked with a fork and ends cut off
- A pinch of sea salt
- ½ cup coconut milk
- ¼ cup coconut, toasted and shredded
- 2 tablespoons cilantro, chopped

Directions:

⇒ In a baking dish, combine all the ingredients, place in the oven at 400 degrees F and bake for 45 minutes.

⇒ Divide between plates and serve.

Nutrition: calories 220, fat 9, fiber 5,3, carbs 33,8, protein 2,6

Chapter 5 -   Snack & Appetizer Recipes

41)Chives Cauliflower Bites

Preparation Time: 5 minutes   **Cooking Time: 30 minutes**   Servings:1

Ingredients:

- 1 small cauliflower head, chopped
- A pinch of sea salt
- ½ teaspoon chives, dried

- ½ teaspoon onion powder
- A drizzle of avocado oil

Directions:

⇒ In a bowl, mix cauliflower popcorn with a pinch of salt and the oil, toss to coat, spread them on a lined baking sheet, and bake at 450 degrees F for 30 minutes, tossing the popcorn halfway.

⇒ Transfer the popcorn to a bowl, add chives and onion powder, stir and serve them.

Nutrition: calories 194, fat 14,3, fiber 6,7, carbs 15, protein 5,4

42)Lemon Cashew Spread

Preparation Time: 10 minutes   **Cooking Time: 0 minutes**   Servings:6

Ingredients:

- ½ cup cashews, soaked for 2 hours and drained
- 1 tablespoon olive oil
- 2 tablespoons lemon juice
- ½ cup pumpkin puree
- 2 tablespoons sesame paste

- 1 garlic clove, minced
- ¼ teaspoon cumin, ground
- A pinch of cayenne pepper
- A pinch of sea salt
- ½ teaspoon pumpkin spice

Directions:

⇒ In your food processor, mix soaked cashews with lemon juice, pumpkin puree, sesame paste, garlic, cumin, pepper, sea salt and pumpkin spice and blend well.

⇒ Add oil gradually, blend again well, transfer to a bowl and serve as a snack.

Nutrition: calories 99, fat 8,2, fiber 1, carbs 5,7, protein 2,2

43)Avocado Dip

Preparation Time: 10 minutes   **Cooking Time: 0 minutes**   Servings:4

Ingredients:

- 3 green onions, chopped
- 3 avocados, pitted, peeled and roughly chopped
- A pinch of pink salt

- 1 teaspoon garlic powder
- Juice of 1 lime

Directions:

⇒ In food processor mix onions with avocados, garlic powder, salt and lime juice and pulse a few times.

⇒ Transfer to a bowl and serve as a snack.

Nutrition: calories 316, fat 29,4, fiber 10,5, carbs 15,2, protein 3,2

44) Lemon Cauliflower Dip

Preparation Time: 10 minutes   **Cooking Time: 40 minutes**   **Servings:4**

Ingredients:

- 4 tablespoons sesame seeds paste
- 1 cauliflower head, florets separated
- 1 small red bell pepper, chopped
- 5 tablespoons olive oil
- 4 tablespoons lemon juice

- 1 teaspoon garlic powder
- Black pepper to taste
- ½ teaspoon cumin, ground
- A pinch of paprika for serving
- A pinch of sea salt

Directions:

⇒ Arrange the cauliflower and bell pepper pieces on a lined baking sheet, drizzle 1 tablespoon over them, toss to coat and bake in the oven at 400 degrees F for 40 minutes.

⇒ Transfer the veggies to a blender, add sesame seeds paste, salt, pepper, the rest of the oil, garlic powder, cumin and lemon juice and blend until you obtain a paste.

⇒ Transfer to a bowl, sprinkle paprika on top and serve as a Paleo snack.

Nutrition: calories 228, fat 22,1, fiber 3,1, carbs 7,9, protein 3,2

45) Tahini Cauliflower Spread

Preparation Time: 10 minutes   **Cooking Time: 45 minutes**   **Servings:6**

Ingredients:

- 1 cauliflower head, florets separated
- ½ cup sun-dried tomatoes, chopped
- 10 garlic cloves
- 4 tablespoons tahini
- 4 tablespoons lemon juice

- 5 tablespoons olive oil
- 1 teaspoon basil, dried
- Black pepper to taste
- 1 teaspoon cumin, ground
- A pinch of sea salt

Directions:

⇒ Put cauliflower florets and garlic cloves on a lined baking sheet, drizzle 1 tablespoon oil over them, toss to coat, place in the oven at 400 degrees F and bake for 45 minutes flipping once.

⇒ Leave cauliflower and garlic to cool down and transfer to a blender.

⇒ Add sun-dried tomatoes, 4 tablespoons oil, black pepper, ½ teaspoon cumin, tahini paste, a pinch of salt and lemon juice and blend until you obtain a paste.

⇒ Transfer to a bowl, sprinkle the rest of the cumin and dried basil on top and serve.

Nutrition: calories 183, fat 17,2, fiber 2,4, carbs 6,9, protein 3,1

46) Lemon Eggplant Hummus

Preparation Time: 10 minutes   **Cooking Time: 1 hour**   **Servings:4**

Ingredients:

- 2 tablespoons lemon juice
- 1 eggplant, cut into halves lengthwise
- 2 tablespoons olive oil

- 1 garlic head, peeled
- Black pepper to the taste
- A pinch of sea salt

Directions:

⇒ Place eggplant halves and the garlic head on a lined baking sheet, drizzle some of the oil over them, place in the oven at 350 degrees F and bake for 1 hour.

⇒ Leave eggplant and garlic to cool down, peel eggplant halves and put everything in your food processor.

⇒ Add a pinch of salt, black pepper, lemon juice and the rest of the oil and pulse well.

⇒ Transfer eggplant spread to a bowl and serve right away.

Nutrition: calories 98, fat 7,3, fiber 4,2, carbs 8,6, protein 1,5

47) Cilantro Egg Bites

Preparation Time: 10 minutes   **Cooking Time: 0 minutes**   **Servings:8**

Ingredients:

- 4 eggs, hard-boiled, peeled and cut in halves
- 1 avocado, pitted, peeled and chopped
- A pinch of sea salt
- Black pepper to taste
- 1 teaspoon cilantro, chopped
- A pinch of garlic powder

Directions:

⇒ Place egg halves on a platter and scoop egg yolks.

⇒ In a bowl, mix egg yolks with avocado, cilantro, a pinch of sea salt, black pepper to the taste and garlic powder.

⇒ Mash everything well and then stuff egg whites with this mix.

⇒ Serve them as an appetizer.

Nutrition: calories 87, fat 7,1, fiber 1,7, carbs 2,3, protein 3,3

48) Turkey Muffins

Preparation Time: 10 minutes   **Cooking Time: 15 minutes**   **Servings:12**

Ingredients:

- A drizzle of avocado oil
- 12 eggs
- 8 asparagus spears, chopped
- A pinch of sea salt
- Black pepper to taste
- 10 ounces turkey meat, cooked, sliced

Directions:

⇒ Divide turkey slices into 12 muffin cups.

⇒ Crack an egg in each, add asparagus pieces on top, season with a pinch of sea salt and black pepper, place in the oven at 400 degrees F and bake for 15 minutes.

⇒ Leave egg cups to cool down, transfer them to a platter and serve.

Nutrition: calories 117, fat 6,7, fiber 0,3, carbs 1, protein 12,8

49) Stuffed Avocado

Preparation Time: 10 minutes   **Cooking Time: 0 minutes**   **Servings:2**

Ingredients:

- 5 ounces cooked salmon
- Juice of 1 lemon
- 1 avocado, pitted and cut in halves
- Black pepper to taste
- 1 tablespoon yellow onion, chopped
- A pinch of sea salt

Directions:

⇒ Scoop most of the avocado flesh and put it in a bowl.

⇒ Add lemon juice, onion, black pepper to the taste, a pinch of salt and salmon, and stir everything very well.

⇒ Stuff the avocado cups with this mix and serve them.

Nutrition: calories 308, fat 24,1, fiber 6,9, carbs 11,2, protein 15,8

Chapter 6 -   Meat Recipes

50) Sage Chicken and Turkey Mix

Preparation Time: 10 minutes   **Cooking Time: 30 minutes**   **Servings:6**

Ingredients:

- 6 chicken thighs, boneless and skinless
- ½ pound turkey meat, cooked, chopped
- 2 tablespoons coconut oil, melted
- A pinch of sea salt

- A handful sage, chopped
- Black pepper to taste
- 3 cups butternut squash, cubed

Directions:

⇒ Heat up a pan over medium heat, add the turkey meat, cook until it's brown, drain on paper towels, transfer to a plate, crumble and leave aside.

⇒ Heat up the same pan over medium heat, add butternut squash, salt and black pepper, stir, cook for 3 minutes, transfer to a plate and leave to one side.

⇒ Heat up the pan again with the coconut oil over medium-high heat, add chicken, salt, and pepper and cook for 10 minutes, turning often.

⇒ Take the pan off the heat, add squash, introduce in the oven at 425 degrees F and bake for 15 minutes.

⇒ Divide chicken and butternut on plates, top with sage and turkey and serve.

Nutrition: calories 401, fat 16,9, fiber 1,4, carbs 8,2, protein 52,3

51) Baked Turkey and Eggplant

Preparation Time: 10 minutes   **Cooking Time: 1 hour**   **Servings:6**

Ingredients:

- 1 sweet potato, chopped
- 1 pound turkey meat, ground
- 1 eggplant, thinly sliced
- 1 yellow onion, chopped
- 1 tablespoon garlic, minced
- A pinch of sea salt
- Black pepper to taste
- ¼ teaspoon chili powder
- ¼ teaspoon cumin, ground
- 10 ounces fresh tomatoes, peeled, chopped

- 8 ounces tomato paste
- A drizzle of olive oil
- ½ teaspoon tarragon, dried

For the sauce:

- 1 tablespoon almond flour
- 1 cup almond milk
- 1 and ½ tablespoons extra virgin olive oil
- 1 tablespoon coconut flour

Directions:

⇒ Heat up a pan over medium-high heat, add turkey meat, onion, and garlic, stir and cook until the meat turns brown.

⇒ Add tomatoes, tomato paste and sweet potatoes, stir and cook for 5 minutes.

⇒ Add a pinch of sea salt, pepper to taste, chili powder, cumin and tarragon, stir well and cook for 2 minutes.

⇒ Grease a baking dish with a drizzle of olive oil, arrange eggplant slices on the bottom and add turkey mix on top.

⇒ Spread turkey mix evenly, introduce dish in the oven at 350 degrees F and bake for 15 minutes.

⇒ Heat up a pot over medium-high heat, add the rest of the olive oil, almond flour and coconut flour, stir well 1 minute, reduce heat, add almond milk, stir and cook for 10 minutes.

⇒ Pour this over the turkey casserole and bake for 45 minutes more.

⇒ Divide between plates and serve.

Nutrition: calories 362, fat 19,2, fiber 7,9, carbs 23,8, protein 27,1

52) Chicken with Broccoli and Sauce

Preparation Time: 15 minutes   **Cooking Time: 20 minutes**   **Servings:4**

Ingredients:

- 1 red bell pepper, chopped
- 1 zucchini, chopped
- 1 yellow onion, finely chopped
- 1 broccoli head, florets separated
- 4 chicken breasts, skinless, boneless and chopped
- A pinch of sea salt
- Black pepper to taste
- 1 tablespoon coconut oil

For the sauce:

- ¼ cup chicken broth
- 2 garlic cloves, minced
- 3 tablespoons coconut amino
- ½ cup orange juice
- 1 tablespoon orange zest, grated
- ¼ teaspoon ginger, grated
- A pinch of red pepper flakes

Directions:

⇒ In a bowl, mix the stock with orange juice, zest, amino, ginger, garlic and the pepper flakes and whisk.

⇒ Heat up a pan with the oil over medium heat, add chicken, cook for 8 minutes and transfer to a plate.

⇒ Heat up the same pan over medium heat, add bell pepper, broccoli florets, onion, and zucchini, stir and cook for 4-5 minutes.

⇒ Add a pinch of sea salt, pepper, orange sauce you've made, stir, bring to a boil, add the chicken, reduce heat and simmer for 8 minutes.

⇒ Divide between plates and serve hot.

Nutrition: calories 574, fat 22,1, fiber 3,6, carbs 16,7, protein 74,6

53) Quail and Grapes Mix

Preparation Time: 15 minutes   **Cooking Time: 1 hour**   **Servings:4**

Ingredients:

- 4 quails
- 1 apple, cored and chopped
- 1 pound green grapes
- 3 small shallots, peeled, sliced
- 1 tablespoon rosemary, chopped
- ½ cup cranberries, chopped

- 2 tablespoons extra virgin olive oil
- 2 garlic cloves, chopped
- 4 rosemary springs, chopped
- ½ cup chicken stock
- A pinch of sea salt
- Black pepper to taste

Directions:

⇒ Pat dry quail, season with sea salt and pepper and leave to one side.

⇒ In a bowl, mix cranberries with chopped rosemary, apple, shallots, olive oil, garlic, salt, and pepper to taste and stir well.

⇒ Stuff quail with this mix, and tie with cooking twine.

⇒ Spread half of the grapes in a baking dish, arrange quail on top, spread the rest of the grapes and pour chicken stock at the end.

⇒ Place everything in the oven at 425 degrees F and bake for 1 hour.

⇒ Divide between plates and serve with baked grapes on the side.

Nutrition: calories 292, fat 11,2, fiber 3,4, carbs 31,8, protein 19,1

54) Orange Duck Mix

Preparation Time: 10 minutes **Cooking Time: 2 hours** **Servings:4**

Ingredients:

- 2 teaspoons allspice, ground
- 4 duck legs
- 4 thyme springs
- 1 lemon, sliced
- 1 orange, sliced

- 1 cup chicken broth
- A pinch of sea salt
- Black pepper to taste
- ½ cup orange juice

Directions:

⇒ Heat up a pan over medium-high heat, add duck legs, season with salt and pepper, and brown them for 3 minutes on each side.

⇒ Arrange half of lemon and orange slices on the bottom of a baking dish, place duck legs, top with the rest of the orange and lemon slices and thyme springs.

⇒ Add chicken stock, orange juice, sprinkle allspice, place in the oven at 350 degrees F and bake for 2 hours.

⇒ Divide between plates and serve hot.

Nutrition: calories 187, fat 5,1, carbs 2, protein 11,3, fiber 24

55) Chicken Balls and Sauce

Preparation Time: 10 minutes **Cooking Time: 20 minutes** **Servings:4**

Ingredients:

- 1 teaspoon sweet paprika
- 1 pineapple, diced
- 1 egg, whisked
- 2 pounds chicken meat, ground
- A pinch of sea salt
- Black pepper to taste
- 1 teaspoon garlic powder
- 1 teaspoon onion powder

For the sauce:

- ¼ cup coconut amino
- 4 tablespoon paleo ketchup
- 1 tablespoon ginger, grated
- ½ cup pineapple juice
- 2 teaspoons raw honey
- ½ teaspoon red pepper flakes
- Salt and black pepper to taste
- 1 tablespoon garlic, minced

Directions:

⇒ In a large saucepan, mix amino with ketchup, ginger, pineapple juice, garlic, pepper flakes, honey, a pinch of sea salt and pepper, stir well, bring to a boil over medium heat, simmer for 8 minutes and take off the heat.

⇒ In a bowl, mix chicken meat with paprika, egg, onion powder, garlic powder, salt and black pepper to taste and stir well.

⇒ Shape meatballs, arrange them on a lined baking sheet, place them in the oven at 475 degrees F and bake for 15 minutes.

⇒ Heat up a pan over medium heat, add pineapple pieces, stir and cook for 2 minutes.

⇒ Add baked meatballs, pour sauce you've made all over, stir gently, cook for 5 minutes, divide between plates and serve.

Nutrition: calories 552, fat 18,3, carbs 1,8, fiber 26,2, protein 68,2

56) Slow Cooked Beef and Onions

Preparation Time: 10 minutes **Cooking Time: 8 hours** Servings:6

Ingredients:

- 2 cups pearl onions
- 3 and ½ pounds grass fed beef meat, cubed
- 4 garlic cloves, minced
- 2 sweet potatoes, chopped
- 2 celery stalks, chopped
- A pinch of sea salt

- Black pepper to taste
- 2 tablespoons tomato paste
- 2 cups carrot, chopped
- 2 cups beef broth
- 1 teaspoon thyme, dried
- 1 tablespoon coconut oil

Directions:

⇒ Heat up a pan with the oil over medium-high heat, add beef, stir and brown for 2 minutes on each side and transfer to a slow cooker.

⇒ Add all the other ingredients, toss, cook on Low for 8 hours, divide between plates and serve.

Nutrition: calories 1689, fat 64,1, fiber 4,2, carbs 23,4, protein 239,1

57) Ginger Lamb

Preparation Time: 10 minutes **Cooking Time: 10 minutes** Servings:6

Ingredients:

- 3 tablespoons coconut aminos
- 4 tablespoons extra virgin olive oil
- 8 lamb chops
- A pinch of sea salt

- Black pepper to taste
- 2 garlic cloves, minced
- 2 tablespoons ginger, minced
- 1 tablespoon parsley leaves, chopped

Directions:

⇒ In a bowl, mix olive oil with coconut amino, garlic, ginger and parsley and stir well.

⇒ Divide lamb chops between plates and serve.

⇒ Season lamb chops with a pinch of sea salt and pepper to taste, place them on preheated grill over medium-high heat and cook for 4 minutes on each side, basting all the time with the marinade.

Nutrition: calories 601, fat 29,4, carbs 2,8, protein 76,8, fiber 0,3

58) Lamb and Squash Mix

Preparation Time: 2 hours **Cooking Time: 1 hour** Servings:4

Ingredients:

- 1 butternut squash, cubed
- 3 pounds lamb shoulder, chopped
- 4 shallots, chopped
- 4 carrots, chopped
- 4 tomatoes, chopped
- 2 Thai chilies, chopped
- 2 tablespoons tomato paste
- 1 cinnamon stick

- 2 and ½ cups warm beef broth
- 1 lemongrass stalk, finely chopped
- 1 teaspoon Chinese five spice powder
- 1 tablespoon ginger, minced
- 2 tablespoon coconut aminos
- 1 and ½ tablespoons coconut oil
- 3 garlic cloves, chopped
- Black pepper to taste

Directions:

⇒ In a bowl, mix lamb with coconut aminos, ginger, lemongrass, garlic and pepper, stir well, cover and keep in the fridge for 2 hours.

⇒ Heat up a pot with the oil over medium-high heat, add marinated lamb, stir and brown for 3 minutes.

⇒ Add tomato paste and tomatoes, stir and cook for 2 more minutes.

⇒ Add squash, shallots, Thai chilies, carrots, cinnamon stick, beef stock and five spices, stir well, place in the oven at 325 degrees F and bake for 1 hour.

⇒ Divide between plates and serve hot.

Nutrition: calories 775, fat 29,6, fiber 33,9, carbs 22,1, protein 100,9

59) Minty Lamb

Preparation Time: 15 minutes   **Cooking Time: 20 minutes**   **Servings:4**

Ingredients:

- 2 garlic cloves, minced
- 8 lamb chops
- 2/3 cup extra virgin olive oil
- 1 tablespoon oregano, finely chopped
- 3 tablespoons Dijon mustard

- 1 tablespoon lemon zest
- 2 tablespoons balsamic vinegar
- 1/3 cup mint, chopped
- Black pepper to taste

Directions:

⇒ In a bowl, mix olive oil with oregano, garlic and lemon zest and stir well.

⇒ Season lamb with black pepper to taste and brush with the mix you've just made.

⇒ Heat up your grill over medium-high heat, add lamb chops, cook for 5 minutes on each side and transfer to plates.

⇒ In a bowl, mix mustard with vinegar, pepper and mint and whisk well.

⇒ Serve lamb chops with vinegar mix drizzled on top.

Nutrition: calories 765, fat 54,3, carbs 1,5, fiber 2,9, protein 63,5

60) Beef and Basil Sauce

Preparation Time: 10 minutes   **Cooking Time: 40 minutes**   **Servings:4**

Ingredients:

- 3 tablespoons Dijon mustard
- 3 pounds beef tenderloin
- A pinch of sea salt
- Black pepper to taste
- 1 tablespoon coconut oil
- 3 tablespoons balsamic vinegar

For the sauce:

- 3 tablespoons basil leaves, chopped

- ½ cup parsley leaves, chopped
- Zest of 1 lemon
- 2 garlic cloves, minced
- A pinch of sea salt
- Black pepper to taste
- ¼ cup extra virgin olive oil

Directions:

⇒ In a bowl, mix mustard with vinegar, stir well and leave to one side.

⇒ Season beef with a pinch of sea salt and pepper to the taste put in a pan heated with the coconut oil over medium-high heat and cook for 2 minutes on each side.

⇒ Transfer beef to a baking pan, cover with the mustard mix, place in the oven at 475 degrees F and bake for 25 minutes.

⇒ In a bowl, mix parsley with basil, lemon zest, garlic, olive oil, a pinch of sea salt, and pepper to taste and whisk very well.

⇒ Take beef tenderloin out of the oven, slice and divide between plates.

⇒ Serve with herbs sauce on the side.

Nutrition: calories 854, fat 47,6, fiber 0,8, carbs 1,8, protein 99,4

61) Beef with Asparagus and Mushrooms

Preparation Time: 10 minutes   **Cooking Time: 20 minutes**   **Servings:4**

Ingredients:

- 10 ounces mushrooms, sliced
- 10 ounces asparagus, sliced
- 1 and ½ pounds beef steak, thinly sliced
- 2 tablespoons coconut sugar
- 1/3 cup coconut amino
- 2 teaspoons apple cider vinegar
- ½ teaspoon ginger, minced
- 6 garlic cloves, minced
- 1 red chili, sliced
- 1 tablespoon coconut oil
- Black pepper to taste

Directions:

⇒ In a bowl, mix garlic with coconut amino, the sugar, ginger and vinegar and whisk well.

⇒ Put some water in a pan, heat up over medium-high heat, add asparagus and black pepper, cook for 3 minutes, transfer to a bowl filled with ice water, drain and leave aside.

⇒ Heat up a pan with the oil over medium-high heat, add mushrooms, cook for 2 minutes on each side, transfer to a bowl and leave aside.

⇒ Heat up the same pan over high heat, add meat, brown for a few minutes and mix with chili pepper.

⇒ Cook for 2 more minutes and mix with asparagus, mushrooms and vinegar sauce you've made at the beginning.

⇒ Stir well, cook for 3 minutes, take off heat, divide between plates and serve.

Nutrition: calories 284, fat 10,4, fiber 2,4, carbs 11,4, protein 36,4

62) Pork and Berry Mix

Preparation Time: 10 minutes   **Cooking Time: 30 minutes**   **Servings:4**

Ingredients:

- 1 cup blueberries
- ½ teaspoon thyme, dried
- 2 pounds pork loin
- 1 tablespoon balsamic vinegar
- ½ teaspoon red chili flakes
- 1 teaspoon ginger powder
- A pinch of sea salt
- Black pepper to taste
- 2 tablespoon water

Directions:

⇒ Put pork loin in a baking dish and season with a pinch of sea salt and pepper to taste.

⇒ Heat up a pan over medium heat, add blueberries and mix with vinegar, water, thyme, chili flakes and ginger.

⇒ Stir well, cook for 5 minutes and pour over pork loin.

⇒ Place in the oven at 375 degrees F and bake for 25 minutes.

⇒ Take pork out of the oven, leave aside for 5 minutes, slice, divide between plates and serve with blueberries sauce.

Nutrition: calories 572, fat 31,7, carbs 5,4, fiber 0,9, protein 62,3

Chapter 7 -   Seafood & Fish Recipes

63) Cilantro Shrimp

Preparation Time: 10 minutes   **Cooking Time: 10 minutes**   **Servings:4**

Ingredients:

- 1 small red bell pepper, chopped
- 1 small yellow onion, chopped
- 20 shrimp, peeled and deveined
- 1 garlic clove, minced
- 1-inch ginger, minced
- ¼ cup coconut aminos
- A pinch of sea salt

- Black pepper to taste
- 2 tablespoons coconut oil
- 2 tablespoons water
- 1 tablespoon lime juice
- 1 teaspoon apple cider vinegar
- A handful cilantro, chopped

Directions:

⇒ In a bowl, mix the aminos with vinegar, water and lime juice and whisk.

⇒ Heat up a pan with the oil over medium heat, add garlic and ginger, stir and cook for 2 minutes.

⇒ Add the onion, bell pepper, stir and cook for 4 minutes.

⇒ Add shrimp, salt, pepper and the vinegar mix, stir and cook for 5 minutes.

⇒ Divide between plates and serve with cilantro sprinkled on top.

Nutrition: calories 218, fat 8,8, carbs 1,1, fiber 8,6, protein 25,9

64) Garlic Halibut Mix

Preparation Time: 10 minutes   **Cooking Time: 15 minutes**   **Servings:4**

Ingredients:

- ¼ cup ghee, melted
- 4 halibut fish fillets, skinless, boneless
- 4 garlic cloves, minced
- 2 tablespoons parsley, chopped

- Zest and juice of 1 lemon
- 1 lemon, sliced
- A pinch of sea salt
- Black pepper to taste

Directions:

⇒ In a bowl, mix the garlic with ghee, lemon zest, juice, parsley, a pinch of sea salt and pepper and whisk.

⇒ Arrange the fish in a baking dish, season with black pepper, drizzle the lemon dressing, top with lemon slices, place in the oven at 425 degrees F and bake for 15 minutes.

⇒ Divide between plates and serve.

Nutrition: calories 1150, fat 62,9, carbs 0,6, fiber 83,5, protein 63

65) Mustard Salmon Mix

Preparation Time: 10 minutes   **Cooking Time: 15 minutes**   **Servings:4**

Ingredients:

- 2 tablespoons pure maple syrup
- 4 salmon fillets, skin on, boneless
- A pinch of sea salt
- White pepper to taste

- 2 teaspoons Dijon mustard
- Juice and zest of 1 orange
- 2 garlic cloves, minced

Directions:

⇒ In a bowl, mix the maple syrup with orange zest, juice, mustard, sea salt, pepper and garlic and whisk well.

⇒ Arrange salmon in a baking dish, brush with the glaze, place in the oven at 400 degrees F and bake for 15 minutes.

⇒ Divide between plates and serve right away.

Nutrition: calories 275, fat 11,2, carbs 0,2, fiber 9,6, protein 34,9

66) Sriracha Lobster

Preparation Time: 10 minutes   **Cooking Time: 10 minutes**   **Servings:4**

Ingredients:

- ¼ cup ghee, melted
- 4 lobster tails
- A pinch of sea salt
- Black pepper to taste

- 2 tablespoons Sriracha sauce
- 1 tablespoon lime juice
- 1 tablespoon chives, chopped
- 1 tablespoon parsley, chopped

Directions:

⇒ In a bowl, mix Sriracha sauce with ghee, chives, salt, pepper and lime juice and whisk well.

⇒ Cut lobster tails halfway through in the center, open them with your fingers, fill them with half of the Sriracha mix, arrange on preheated grill over medium-high heat, cook for 4 minutes, flip and cook for 3 minutes more.

⇒ Divide lobster tails between plates, drizzle the rest of the Sriracha sauce, sprinkle parsley on top and serve.

Nutrition: calories 245, fat 14 carbs 1, fiber 0,1, protein 27,7

67) Garlic Clams

Preparation Time: 10 minutes   **Cooking Time: 10 minutes**   **Servings:2**

Ingredients:

- 3 tablespoons ghee
- 1 and ½ pounds shell clams, scrubbed
- 1 cup chicken stock
- 3 garlic cloves, minced

- A pinch of sea salt
- Black pepper to taste
- 2 tablespoons parsley, chopped

Directions:

⇒ Heat up a large saucepan with the ghee over medium heat, add garlic, stir and cook for 1 minute.

⇒ Add the stock and clams, bring to a boil, cover the pot and cook for 4-5 minutes.

⇒ Divide the mix into bowls, sprinkle the parsley on top, salt and pepper and serve.

Nutrition: calories 306, fat 19,4, carbs 0,2, fiber 7,2, protein 25,8

68) Coconut Salmon Mix

Preparation Time: 15 minutes   **Cooking Time: 1 hour and 10 minutes**   **Servings:4**

Ingredients:

- 8 sweet potatoes, thinly sliced
- 4 cups salmon meat, cooked and shredded
- 1 red onion, chopped
- 2 carrots, chopped
- 1 celery stalk, chopped
- A pinch of sea salt

- Black pepper to taste
- 2 tablespoons chives, chopped
- 2 cups coconut milk
- 2 garlic cloves, minced
- 3 tablespoons ghee

Directions:

⇒ Heat up a pan with the ghee over medium heat, add the garlic, stir and cook for 1 minute.

⇒ Add coconut milk, salt and pepper, stir, cook for 3 minutes more and take off the heat.

⇒ In a bowl, mix the carrots with salmon, celery, chives, onion and pepper to taste and stir.

⇒ Arrange a layer of potatoes in a baking dish, add some of the coconut sauce, add half of the salmon mix, the rest of the potatoes, top with the remaining sauce, place in the oven at 375 degrees F and bake for 1 hour.

⇒ Divide between plates and serve hot.

Nutrition: calories 921, fat 40,7, carbs 96,6, fiber 16,4, protein 48,1

69) Citrus Calamari Mix

Preparation Time: 10 minutes   **Cooking Time: 5 minutes**   **Servings:4**

Ingredients:

- 2 pounds calamari, tentacles and tubes sliced into rings
- 1 lime, sliced
- 1 lemon, sliced
- 1 orange, sliced
- 2 tablespoons parsley, chopped
- A pinch of sea salt
- Black pepper to taste
- 3 tablespoons lemon juice
- ¼ cup extra virgin olive oil
- 2 garlic cloves, minced

Directions:

⇒ In a bowl, mix calamari with sliced lemon, lime, orange, lemon juice, a pinch of sea salt, pepper, parsley, garlic and olive oil and toss to coat.

⇒ Heat up your kitchen grill over medium-high heat, add calamari rings, lemon, lime and orange slices, cook for 5 minutes, divide between plates and serve.

Nutrition: calories 1108, fat 48,9, carbs 85,9, fiber 6,6, protein 73

70) Chives Shrimp and Zucchini Mix

Preparation Time: 10 minutes   **Cooking Time: 15 minutes**   **Servings:2**

Ingredients:

- 2 zucchinis, cut with a spiralizer
- 1 pound shrimp, peeled and deveined
- 4 garlic cloves, minced
- A pinch of sea salt
- Black pepper to taste
- ¼ cup chicken stock
- 2 tablespoons chives, chopped
- 2 tablespoons lemon juice
- 2 tablespoons coconut oil, melted

Directions:

⇒ Heat up a pan with the oil over medium-high heat, add the garlic, stir and cook for 3 minutes.

⇒ Add shrimp, stir and cook for 3 minutes and transfer them to a plate.

⇒ Pour lemon juice and the stock into the pan, bring to a boil over medium heat and simmer for 5 minutes.

⇒ Add zucchini noodles, the shrimp, salt and pepper, stir gently, divide between plates, sprinkle chives on top and serve.

Nutrition: calories 433, fat 18, carbs 2,4, fiber 12,5, protein 54,7

71) Scallops and Cauliflower Mix

Preparation Time: 10 minutes   **Cooking Time: 25 minutes**   **Servings:4**

Ingredients:

- 3 garlic cloves, minced
- 2 cups cauliflower florets, chopped
- 2 cups sweet potatoes, chopped
- 2 rosemary springs
- 12 sea scallops
- A pinch of sea salt
- Black pepper to taste
- ¼ cup pine nuts, toasted
- 2 cups veggie stock
- 2 tablespoons olive oil
- A handful chives, chopped

Directions:

⇒ Put cauliflower, potatoes and the stock in a large saucepan, bring to a boil over medium-high heat, reduce temperature and simmer for 20 minutes.

⇒ Drain veggies, transfer them to a blender, add salt and pepper and pulse well.

⇒ Heat up a pan with the oil over medium-high heat, add rosemary and garlic, stir and cook for 1 minute.

⇒ Add scallops, cook them for 2 minutes, season them with pepper to the taste and take them off the heat.

⇒ Divide the puree between plates, arrange scallops on top, sprinkle chives and pine nuts at the end and serve.

Nutrition: calories 308, fat 14,8, fiber 4,9, carbs 28,8, protein 18,6

72) Chili Salmon Mix

Preparation Time: 20 minutes   **Cooking Time: 10 minutes**   **Servings:4**

Ingredients:

- 1 teaspoon cumin, ground
- 1 teaspoon sweet paprika
- 1 teaspoon chili powder
- 1 teaspoon onion powder
- ½ teaspoon garlic powder
- 4 salmon fillets, boneless
- A pinch of sea salt
- Black pepper to taste

For the avocado sauce:

- 2 avocados, pitted, peeled and chopped
- 1 garlic clove, minced
- Juice of 1 lime
- 1 red onion, chopped
- 1 tablespoon olive oil
- Black pepper to taste
- 1 tablespoon cilantro, finely chopped

Directions:

⇒ In a bowl, mix paprika with cumin, onion powder, garlic powder, chili powder, salt, pepper and the salmon, toss and keep in the fridge for 20 minutes.

⇒ Put avocado in a bowl, mash well with a fork, add red onion, garlic clove, lime juice, olive oil, chopped cilantro, and pepper to taste and stir.

⇒ Put the salmon on preheated grill over medium-high heat, cook for 3 minutes on each side and divide between plates.

⇒ Top each salmon piece with avocado sauce and serve.

Nutrition: calories 494, fat 34,4, carbs 14, fiber 7,9, protein 37,2

73) Tilapia Tortillas

Preparation Time: 15 minutes   **Cooking Time: 10 minutes**   **Servings:4**

Ingredients:

- 1 pound tilapia fillets, boneless, skinless and cubed
- ¼ cup coconut flour
- 2 eggs
- ¼ cup sparkling water
- 2 cups green cabbage, shredded
- 2 cups coconut oil, melted
- A pinch of sea salt and black pepper
- Lime wedges for serving
- 4 cauliflower tortillas

For the Pico de Gallo:

- 2 tomatoes, chopped
- 2 tablespoons jalapeno, chopped
- 6 tablespoons yellow onion, chopped
- 2 tablespoons lime juice
- 1 tablespoon cilantro, chopped

For the mayonnaise sauce:

- ¼ cup homemade mayonnaise
- 2 teaspoons lime juice

Directions:

⇒ In a bowl, mix tomatoes with the onion, jalapeno, cilantro, 2 tablespoons lime juice, toss, cover and keep in the fridge.

⇒ In another bowl, mix the mayo with 2 teaspoons lime juice, whisk, cover and keep in the fridge.

⇒ In a bowl, mix the coconut flour with sparkling water, a pinch of sea salt, pepper and eggs and whisk very well.

⇒ Pat dry fish cubes and dredge them in eggs mix.

⇒ Heat up a pan with the coconut oil over medium-high heat, add fish cubes, cook for 2 minutes on each side, transfer to paper towels and drain excess fat.

⇒ Arrange tortillas on a working surface, divide the cabbage and the fish on each, add some of the Pico de Gallo and top with mayo.

⇒ Serve with lime wedges on the side.

Nutrition: calories 1256, fat 119,2, carbs 31,5, fiber 8,6, protein 28,3

74) Smoked Salmon Salad

Preparation Time: 10 minutes   **Cooking Time: 0 minutes**   **Servings:2**

Ingredients:

- 2 cups cherry tomatoes, halved
- 1 red onion, thinly sliced
- 8 ounces smoked salmon, cut into thin slices
- 1 cucumber, thinly chopped
- 6 tablespoons extra virgin olive oil
- ½ teaspoon garlic, minced

- 2 tablespoons lemon juice
- Black pepper to taste
- 1 teaspoon balsamic vinegar
- 1 tablespoon dill, chopped
- ½ teaspoon oregano, dried

Directions:

⇒ In a bowl, mix the oil with garlic, balsamic vinegar, oregano, black pepper and the garlic and whisk well.

⇒ In a bowl, mix the cucumber with tomatoes and onion, drizzle the dressing over veggies and toss to coat.

⇒ Roll salmon pieces and divide them between plates.

⇒ Add mixed veggies on the side, sprinkle dill all over and serve.

Nutrition: calories 580, fat 47,7, carbs 19,3, fiber 4,5, protein 24,4

75) Dill Trout

Preparation Time: 10 minutes   **Cooking Time: 20 minutes**   **Servings:4**

Ingredients:

- 3 trout, cleaned and gutted
- 1 bunch dill
- 2 lemons, sliced
- 1 bunch rosemary

- 2 fennel bulbs, sliced
- A pinch of sea salt
- Black pepper to taste
- 2 tablespoons extra virgin olive oil

Directions:

⇒ Grease a baking dish with some oil, spread fennel slices on the bottom, add the trout and season with salt and pepper.

⇒ Stuff each fish with lemon slices, dill and rosemary springs, top the fish with the rest of the herbs and lemon slices, drizzle the rest of the oil, place everything in the oven at 500 degrees F and bake for 10 minutes.

⇒ Reduce heat to 425 degrees F and bake for 12 more minutes.

⇒ Leave fish to cool down, divide between plates and serve.

Nutrition: calories 279, fat 15,3, carbs 9,7, fiber 4,2, protein 26,6

76) Lemon Cod

Preparation Time: 10 minutes   **Cooking Time: 20 minutes**   **Servings:4**

Ingredients:

- ¼ cup ghee
- 4 medium cod fillets, skinless
- 2 garlic cloves, minced
- 1 tablespoon parsley, finely chopped
- 1 teaspoon mustard
- 1 shallot, chopped

- 2 tablespoons lemon juice
- 2 tablespoons coconut oil, melted
- A pinch of sea salt
- Black pepper to taste
- Lemon wedges for serving

Directions:

⇒ In a bowl, mix parsley with ghee, mustard, garlic, shallot, a pinch of sea salt, pepper and lemon juice and whisk very well.

⇒ Heat up an oven proof pan with the coconut oil over medium-high heat, add fish, season with black pepper to the taste and cook for 4 minutes on each side.

⇒ Spread ghee mix over fish, place in the oven at 425 degrees F and bake for 10 minutes.

⇒ Divide between plates and serve with lemon wedges on the side.

Nutrition: calories 275, fat 20,9, carbs 2,4, fiber 0,3, protein 20,7

Chapter 8 -   Salad Recipes

77) Veggie and Eggs Salad

Preparation Time: 10 minutes   **Cooking Time: 10 minutes**   **Servings:4**

Ingredients:

- 1 avocado, pitted, peeled and chopped
- 1 small red onion, chopped
- 4 eggs
- 1 small red bell pepper, chopped

- ¼ cup homemade mayonnaise
- A pinch of sea salt
- Black pepper to taste
- 1 tablespoon lemon juice

Directions:

⇒ Put eggs in a large saucepan, add water to cover, place on stove over medium-high heat, bring to a boil, reduce heat to low and cook for 10 minutes.

⇒ Drain eggs, leave them in cold water to cool down, peel, chop them and put in a salad bowl.

⇒ Add a pinch of sea salt and pepper to taste, onion, bell pepper, avocado, lemon juice and mayo, toss to coat and serve right away.

Nutrition: calories 240, fat 19,2, carbs 12,1, fiber 4,2, protein 7,1

78) Tomato and Pear Bowl

Preparation Time: 10 minutes   **Cooking Time:**   **Servings:4**

Ingredients:

- 1 pear, sliced
- 5 cups lettuce leaves, torn
- 1 small cucumber, chopped
- ½ cup cherry tomatoes, cut in halves
- ½ cup red grapes, cut in halves
- A pinch of sea salt

- Black pepper to taste
- 3 tablespoons orange juice
- ¼ cup extra virgin olive oil
- 1 tablespoon orange zest, grated
- 1 tablespoon parsley, minced

Directions:

⇒

⇒ In a bowl, mix all the ingredients, toss, divide between plates and serve.

Nutrition: calories 174, fat 12,9, carbs 16,2, fiber 2,5, protein 1,4

79) Tomato and Seafood Salad

Preparation Time: 20 minutes   **Cooking Time: 10 minutes**   **Servings:2**

Ingredients:

- 5 cups mixed greens
- ½ cup cherry tomatoes, cut in halves
- 1 pound shrimp, peeled and deveined
- 1 small red onion, thinly sliced
- 1 avocado, pitted, peeled and chopped
- Black pepper to taste

- ½ tablespoon sweet paprika
- ½ teaspoon cumin
- 1 tablespoon chili powder
- 1/3 cup cilantro, finely chopped
- ½ cup lime juice
- ¼ cup extra virgin olive oil

Directions:

⇒ In a bowl, mix chili powder with cumin, paprika, ¼ cup lime juice and shrimp, toss to coat and leave aside for 20 minutes.

⇒ Place shrimps under preheated broiler on medium-high heat, cook for 4 minutes on each side and transfer to a bowl.

⇒ In a small bowl, mix cilantro with oil, the rest of the lime juice and pepper to taste and whisk well.

⇒ In a large salad bowl, mix greens with tomatoes, onion, avocado and shrimp.

⇒ Add salad dressing, toss to coat and serve right away.

Nutrition: calories 1028, fat 50,4, carbs 80, fiber 30,1, protein 68,2

80) Tomato and Greens Salad

Preparation Time: 10 minutes   **Cooking Time: 8 minutes**   **Servings:4**

Ingredients:

- ½ cup sun-dried tomatoes, sliced
- 1 eggplant, sliced
- 1 green onion, sliced
- Black pepper to taste
- 4 cups mixed salad greens
- 1 tablespoon mint leaves, finely chopped
- 1 tablespoon oregano, finely chopped
- 1 tablespoon parsley leaves, finely chopped
- 4 tablespoons extra virgin olive oil

For the salad dressing:

- 2 garlic cloves, minced
- ¼ cup extra virgin olive oil
- ½ tablespoon mustard
- 1 tablespoon lemon juice
- ½ teaspoon smoked paprika
- A pinch of sea salt
- Black pepper to the taste

Directions:

⇒ Brush eggplant slices with olive oil, season with black pepper, place them under a preheated broiler on medium-high heat, cook for 3 minutes on each side and transfer them to a salad bowl.

⇒ Add sun-dried tomatoes, onion, greens, mint, parsley, oregano and pepper to taste and 4 tablespoons olive oil and toss to coat.

⇒ In a small bowl, mix ¼ cup olive oil with garlic, mustard, paprika, lemon juice, salt, and pepper to taste and whisk very well.

⇒ Pour this over salad, toss to coat gently and serve.

Nutrition: calories 179, fat 13,6, carbs 14,5, fiber 5,4, protein 3,8

81) Chili Potato and Shallots Salad

Preparation Time: 15 minutes   **Cooking Time: 30 minutes**   **Servings:4**

Ingredients:

- 8 sweet potatoes, chopped
- 1 tablespoon coriander seeds
- 1 teaspoon cumin seeds
- 1 red onion, sliced
- ½ tablespoon oregano, dried
- A pinch of sea salt
- Black pepper to taste

- 3 small shallots, peeled, chopped, already cooked
- ½ teaspoon chili flakes
- ¼ cup extra virgin olive oil
- 3 tablespoons parsley, chopped
- 1 tablespoon coconut oil
- 2 tablespoons balsamic vinegar

Directions:

⇒ Put potatoes in a large saucepan, add water to cover, bring to a boil over medium-high heat, cook for 20 minutes, drain water and put them in a bowl.

⇒ Heat up a pan with the coconut oil over medium-high heat, add onions, stir, reduce temperature to low, cook for 10 minutes and transfer them to a bowl.

⇒ Return pan to medium-high heat, add cumin seeds and coriander seeds, stir, toast for 2 minutes and add them to the bowl with the onions.

⇒ Also add chili flakes, oregano, shallots, parsley, olive oil, vinegar, a pinch of sea salt and pepper to taste and stir everything well.

⇒ Add potatoes, toss to coat and serve cold.

Nutrition: calories 521, fat 16,8, carbs 90, fiber 13,3, protein 5,6

82) Chicken and Pineapple Salad

Preparation Time: 10 minutes   **Cooking Time: 50 minutes**   **Servings:4**

Ingredients:

- 2 chicken breasts, skinless and boneless
- 1 pineapple, peeled and sliced
- 6 cups mixed salad greens
- 1 red onion, sliced
- ¼ cup pineapple sauce
- ½ cup cherry tomatoes, halved
- A pinch of sea salt
- Black pepper to taste
- ¼ cup extra virgin olive oil
- 2 tablespoons apple cider vinegar

For the sauce:

- 1 yellow onion, minced
- 1 garlic clove, minced
- 6 ounces tomato paste
- ½ cup apple cider vinegar
- ½ cup water
- ¼ cup paleo ketchup
- 3 tablespoons mustard
- 1 pinch cloves, ground
- A pinch of cinnamon
- A pinch of smoked paprika

Directions:

⇒ Heat up a pan over medium-high heat, add 1 yellow onion, stir and brown for 3 minutes.

⇒ Add garlic and cook 1 more minute.

⇒ Add tomato paste, ½ cup vinegar, water, ketchup, mustard, cloves, cinnamon and a pinch of smoked paprika, stir everything well, bring to a boil, reduce heat to medium-low and simmer for 30 minutes.

⇒ Take sauce off heat, reserve 1 cup and keep the rest in the fridge for another occasion.

⇒ Season chicken breast with a pinch of sea salt and pepper to taste, place them under a preheated broiler on medium-high heat, cook for 8 minutes on each side.

⇒ Brush chicken with 1 cup of the sauce you've just made and cook for 4 more minutes on each side.

⇒ Transfer chicken to a cutting board, leave aside to cool down, slice and put in a salad bowl.

⇒ Grill pineapple on medium-high heat, transfer to a cutting board as well, cut into small cubes and add to chicken.

⇒ Also add greens, red onion, grape tomatoes and pepper to taste.

⇒ In a small bowl, mix pineapple juice with 2 tablespoons vinegar, ¼ cup olive oil, a pinch of sea salt and pepper to taste and stir well.

⇒ Pour this over chicken salad, toss to coat and serve.

Nutrition: calories 554, fat 23,7, carbs 49,9, fiber 5,1, protein 39,6

83) Chicken and Berries Salad

Preparation Time: 10 minutes   **Cooking Time: 15 minutes**   **Servings:2**

Ingredients:

- 2 teaspoons parsley, dried
- 2 chicken breasts, skinless and boneless
- ½ teaspoon onion powder
- ½ cup lemon juice
- 2 teaspoons paprika
- A pinch of sea salt
- Black pepper to taste

- 8 strawberries, sliced
- 1 small red onion, sliced
- 6 cups baby spinach
- 1 avocado, peeled and cut into small chunks
- ¼ cup extra virgin olive oil
- 1 tablespoon tarragon, chopped
- 2 tablespoons balsamic vinegar

Directions:

⇒ Put chicken in a bowl, add lemon juice, parsley, onion powder and paprika and toss to coat.

⇒ Place chicken under a preheated broiler on medium-high heat, cook for 10 minutes on each side, transfer to a cutting board and slice.

⇒ In a bowl, mix oil with vinegar, a pinch of sea salt, pepper and tarragon and whisk well.

⇒ In a salad bowl, mix spinach with onion, avocado, and strawberry.

⇒ Add chicken pieces and the vinaigrette, toss to coat and serve.

Nutrition: calories 916, fat 62,4, carbs 22,5, fiber 11,6, protein 69,7

84) Lemon Radish and Cucumber Salad

Preparation Time: 10 minutes   **Cooking Time: 0 minutes**   **Servings:4**

Ingredients:

- 8 radishes, sliced
- 1 cucumber, sliced
- 1 apple, chopped
- 1 celery stalk, chopped
- Black pepper to taste

- ¼ cup homemade mayonnaise
- 2 tablespoons chives, chopped
- 2 tablespoons apple cider vinegar
- 2 tablespoons lemon juice

Directions:

⇒ In a bowl, mix radishes with apple, celery, and cucumber.

⇒ In a small bowl, mix mayo with vinegar, pepper, lemon juice and chives and whisk well.

⇒ Pour this over salad, toss to coat and keep in the fridge until you serve it.

Nutrition: calories 104, fat 5,2, carbs 14,7, fiber 2, protein 1

85) Sprouts and Cabbage Salad

Preparation Time: 10 minutes   **Cooking Time: 0 minutes**   **Servings:4**

Ingredients:

- 4 cups Brussels sprouts
- 2 cups red cabbage, shredded
- Black pepper to taste
- 1 red apple, sliced
- 2 celery stalks, chopped

- 2 tablespoons lemon juice
- ¼ cup walnuts, chopped
- ¼ cup homemade mayonnaise
- 4 tablespoons apple cider vinegar

Directions:

⇒ In a bowl, combine all the ingredients, toss, divide between plates and serve.

⇒

Nutrition: calories 188, fat 10, carbs 22,6, fiber 6,2, protein 5,7

86) Lime Veggie Noodle Salad

Preparation Time: 15 minutes   **Cooking Time:0**   **Servings:4**

Ingredients:

- 3 carrots, thinly sliced with a spiralizer
- 2 cucumbers, thinly sliced with a spiralizer
- 1 green onion, sliced
- 1 tablespoon sesame seeds
- 2 tablespoons lime juice

- A pinch of sea salt
- 2 tablespoons balsamic vinegar
- Black pepper to taste
- 2 tablespoons extra virgin olive oil

Directions:

⇒ In a salad bowl, mix cucumbers with green onion and carrots.

⇒ In a small bowl, mix vinegar with olive oil, lime juice, a pinch of sea salt, and pepper to taste and stir well.

⇒ Pour this over salad, toss to coat and keep in the fridge until you serve it.

Nutrition: calories 117, fat 8,3, carbs 11,2, fiber 2,3, protein 1,9

87) Greens and Orange Salad

Preparation Time: 15 minutes   **Cooking Time: 0 minutes**   Servings:4

Ingredients:

- 1 avocado, pitted, peeled and chopped
- 8 cups mixed salad greens
- 2 tablespoons pine nuts, toasted
- 6 figs, cut into quarters
- ¾ cup pomegranate seeds
- 2 oranges, peeled and cut into segments
- ¼ cup extra virgin olive oil

- 1 tablespoon lemon juice
- 4 tablespoons orange juice
- 2 tablespoons white wine vinegar
- 1 teaspoon orange zest
- A pinch of sea salt
- Black pepper to taste

Directions:

⇒ In a salad bowl, mix greens with avocado, figs, oranges, pine nuts and pomegranate seeds.

⇒ In another bowl, mix orange juice with lemon juice, olive oil, orange zest, vinegar, a pinch of sea salt and pepper to taste and whisk well.

⇒ Pour this over salad, toss to coat and serve.

Nutrition: calories 427, fat 26, carbs 49,2, fiber 8,8, protein 7,2

88) Lobster, Grapefruit and Greens Salad

Preparation Time: 10 minutes   **Cooking Time: 0 minutes**   Servings:2

Ingredients:

- 1 grapefruit, peeled and chopped
- 1 pound lobster meat, cooked and chopped
- 1 avocado, pitted, peeled and chopped
- 1 shallot, chopped
- 3 cups mixed greens
- 2 tablespoons grapefruit juice

- 1 tablespoon chives, chopped
- A pinch of sea salt
- Black pepper to taste
- 4 tablespoons extra virgin olive oil
- 2 tablespoons balsamic vinegar
- Some dill, finely chopped for serving

Directions:

⇒ In a bowl, mix grapefruit juice with oil, vinegar, chives, shallot, a pinch of sea salt and pepper to taste and stir very well.

⇒ Add lobster meat and toss to coat.

⇒ In a large bowl, mix avocado with greens and grapefruit.

⇒ Add lobster meat and dressing on top, sprinkle dill all over and serve.

Nutrition: calories 860, fat 50, carbs 52,3, fiber 19,5, protein 53,6

89) Ginger Steak and Veggie Salad

Preparation Time: 1 hour   **Cooking Time: 15 minutes**   **Servings:4**

Ingredients:

- 4 cups lettuce leaves, torn
- 1 pound steak
- 1 red bell pepper, cut into strips
- 1 cucumber, sliced
- ¼ cup mint leaves, chopped
- ¼ cup cilantro, chopped
- 1 tablespoon ginger, grated
- ¼ cup coconut aminos
- 1 Thai red chili pepper, chopped
- 3 garlic cloves, minced
- Juice from 1 lime

- A pinch of sea salt
- Black pepper to taste
- Silvered almonds for serving
- For the salad dressing:
- 3 tablespoons coconut aminos
- 2 tablespoons melted coconut oil
- 1 teaspoon fish sauce
- Zest of 1 lime
- Juice of 1 lime
- 1 Thai red chili pepper, chopped

Directions:

⇒ In a bowl, mix garlic with ginger, 1 red chili, juice from 1 lime and ¼ cup coconut aminos and stir.

⇒ Add steak, toss to coat, cover bowl and keep in the fridge for 1 hour.

⇒ In another bowl, mix 2 tablespoons coconut oil with 3 tablespoons coconut aminos, 1 lime chili pepper, fish sauce, zest and juice from 1 lime, stir well and leave aside for now.

⇒ Place steak under preheated broiler on medium-high heat, cook for 4 minutes on each side, transfer to a cutting board, leave aside for 4 minutes, slice very thinly and put in a salad bowl.

⇒ Add lettuce, cucumber, bell pepper, a pinch of sea salt and pepper to taste. Add salad dressing you've made, toss to coat, sprinkle cilantro, mint, and almonds and serve.

Nutrition: calories 312, fat 9,9, carbs 10,9, fiber 1,9, protein 42,8

90) Tomato and Olives Salad

Preparation Time: 15 minutes   **Cooking Time: 0 minutes**   **Servings:4**

Ingredients:

- 1 cucumber, chopped
- 4 medium tomatoes, chopped
- 1 red onion, sliced
- 1 green bell pepper, chopped
- ¾ cup kalamata olives, pitted and chopped

- 1 tablespoon lemon juice
- ¼ cup extra virgin olive oil
- ½ teaspoon oregano, dried
- 2 tablespoons balsamic vinegar
- Black pepper to taste

Directions:

⇒ In a small bowl, mix lemon juice with oil, oregano, vinegar and pepper to taste and whisk well.

⇒ In a salad bowl, mix tomatoes with bell pepper, onion, and cucumber.

⇒ Add salad dressing, toss to coat and serve with olives on top.

Nutrition: calories 194, fat 15,8, carbs 14,2, fiber 2,8, protein 3,4

Chapter 9 -   Dessert Recipes

91) Cocoa Balls

Preparation Time: 30 minutes   **Cooking Time: 0 minute**   **Servings:4**

Ingredients:

- 10 hazelnuts, roasted
- 1 cup hazelnuts, roasted and chopped
- 1 teaspoon vanilla extract

- 2 tablespoons raw cocoa powder
- ¼ cup maple syrup

Directions:

⇒ Put ½ cup chopped hazelnuts in a food processor and blend well.

⇒ Add vanilla extract, cocoa powder, and maple syrup and blend again.

⇒ Roll the 10 hazelnuts in cocoa powder mix, dip them in the rest of the chopped hazelnuts and arrange balls on a lined baking sheet.

⇒ Place in the freezer for 20 minutes and then serve them.

Nutrition: calories 378, fat 31,2, carbs 23,3, fiber 5,7, protein 8,1

92) Almond Cookies

Preparation Time: 10 minutes   **Cooking Time: 20 minutes**   **Servings:4**

Ingredients:

- ¼ cup apple sauce
- 1 and ½ cup pumpkin puree
- 1 teaspoon vanilla extract
- ¼ cup coconut milk

- 1 cup almond milk
- ½ teaspoon pumpkin pie spice
- ½ cup coconut flour

Directions:

⇒ In a bowl, mix applesauce with pumpkin puree, vanilla extract, and coconut milk and stir very well.

⇒ Add almond meal, pumpkin pie spice, and coconut flour and stir well again.

⇒ Drop spoonfuls of batter on a lined baking sheet, flatten with a fork, place in the oven at 350 degrees F and bake for 25 minutes.

⇒ Take cookies out of the oven, leave aside to cool down, transfer to a platter and serve.

Nutrition: calories 351, fat 21,9, carbs 34,8, fiber 18,8, protein 7,4

93) Maple Berry Bars

Preparation Time: 30 minutes   **Cooking Time: 7 minutes**   **Servings:9**

Ingredients:

- ½ cup coconut butter
- ¾ cup melted coconut oil
- ¾ cup cocoa powder
- 1 tablespoon cocoa butter

- ½ cup maple syrup
- ½ cup raspberries
- ¼ cup almonds, roasted and chopped

Directions:

⇒ Heat up a pan over medium heat, add coconut oil, coconut butter, maple syrup, cocoa butter, and cocoa powder and stir well until everything blends.

⇒ Add almonds, and raspberries and stir again.

⇒ Pour this mix into a lined baking tray, place in the freezer for 20 minutes, slice, arrange on plates and serve.

Nutrition: calories 221, fat 16,9, carbs 20,2, fiber 5,1, protein 2,8

94) Cocoa Muffins

Preparation Time: 10 minutes   **Cooking Time: 30 minutes**   **Servings:8**

Ingredients:

- 1 cup almond butter
- 1 egg, whisked
- 3 bananas, chopped

- ½ cup cocoa powder
- 2 tablespoons raw honey
- 2 teaspoons vanilla extract

Directions:

⇒ In a bowl, mix almond butter with bananas, cocoa powder, egg, vanilla extract and honey and stir well.

⇒ Pour this into a muffin tray, place in the oven at 375 degrees F and bake for 30 minutes.

⇒ Leave muffins to cool down for 5 minutes, removed from muffin tray and serve.

Nutrition: calories 90, fat 2,5, carbs 17,9, fiber 3, protein 2,6

95) Lemon Baked Apples

Preparation Time: 10 minutes   **Cooking Time: 40 minutes**   **Servings:4**

Ingredients:

- 4 apples, peeled
- 1 cup fresh blueberries
- 2 teaspoons lemon juice
- ½ cup apple juice

- ½ teaspoon cinnamon, ground
- 4 tablespoons almond meal
- 4 tablespoons coconut flakes

Directions:

⇒ Scoop the inside of each apple, brush them with lemon juice and place in a baking dish.

⇒ Fill apples with blueberries and sprinkle cinnamon on top.

⇒ Spread the rest of the blueberries in the baking dish, pour apple juice, sprinkle almond meal and coconut flakes on each apple, place everything in the oven at 375 degrees F and bake for 40 minutes.

⇒ Take apples out of the oven, leave them to cool down, divide between plates and serve.

Nutrition: calories 204, fat 5,2, carbs 41,9, fiber 7,7, protein 2,4

96) Berry Popsicles

Preparation Time: 2 hours   **Cooking Time: 15 minutes**   **Servings:4**

Ingredients:

- 1 and ½ cups raspberries

- 2 cups water

Directions:

⇒ Put raspberries and water in a saucepan, heat up over medium heat, bring to a boil and simmer for 15 minutes.

⇒ Take off heat, pour the mix into an ice cube tray, add a popsicle stick in each, introduce in the freezer and chill for 2 hours.

Nutrition: calories 23, fat 0,2, carbs 0, fiber 0, protein 0

97) Spiced Pudding

Preparation Time: 10 minutes   **Cooking Time: 8 minutes**   **Servings:4**

Ingredients:

- 1 and ¾ cup almond milk
- ½ cup pumpkin puree
- 2 tablespoons coconut flour
- ¼ cup stevia
- 1 tablespoon water
- 1 egg
- 1 teaspoon vanilla extract
- ¼ teaspoon nutmeg, ground
- ½ teaspoon cinnamon, ground
- 1/8 teaspoon allspice, ground
- ¼ teaspoon ginger, ground

Directions:

⇒ In a bowl, mix coconut flour with water and stir well.

⇒ Put almond milk in a saucepan and mix with the stevia and egg.

⇒ Stir, bring to a boil and stir in the coconut mix.

⇒ Cook for 2 minutes and take off heat.

⇒ In a bowl, mix pumpkin puree with vanilla extract, nutmeg, cinnamon, allspice and ginger and stir well.

⇒ Pour this into almond milk mix, stir and place over medium-high heat.

⇒ Cook for 4 minutes, transfer to dessert bowls and serve after you've chilled in the freezer for 2 hours.

Nutrition: calories 108, fat 4,1, carbs 24,1, fiber 3,2, protein 3,4

98) Coconut and Banana Pancakes

Preparation Time: 15 minutes   **Cooking Time: 20 minutes**   **Servings:4**

Ingredients:

- ¼ cup coconut milk
- 1 banana, peeled and mashed
- 4 eggs
- 1 teaspoon vanilla extract
- 1 and ½ cups hazelnut meal
- 2 tablespoons coconut flour
- ½ teaspoon baking soda
- Ghee for cooking

For the sauce:

- 2 tablespoons coconut oil
- 1 tablespoon lemon juice
- 2 blood oranges, peeled and sliced
- Juice from 1 blood orange
- 2 teaspoons stevia
- 1 vanilla bean

Directions:

⇒ Heat up a pan with the coconut oil over medium heat, add orange juice, lemon juice, stevia and vanilla bean, bring to a boil and simmer for 15 minutes stirring from time to time.

⇒ In a bowl, mix eggs with vanilla extract and coconut milk and stir.

⇒ Add mashed banana, coconut flour, baking soda and hazelnut meal and stir well.

⇒ Heat up a pan with the ghee over medium heat, spoon ¼ cup pancake mix, spread a bit, cook for 3 minutes on one side, flip, cook for 1 more minute and transfer to a plate.

⇒ Repeat this with the rest of the batter and serve pancakes with orange slices on the side and with the orange sauce on top.

Nutrition: calories 696, fat 56,5, carbs 41,4, fiber 12,7, protein 17

99) Cherry Bowls

Preparation Time: 10 minutes   **Cooking Time: 40 minutes**   **Servings:4**

Ingredients:

- 1 cup stevia
- 1 tablespoon lemon juice
- 6 cups cherries, pitted and roughly chopped

Directions:

⇒ Put cherries in a pan, add the stevia and leave aside for 10 minutes.

⇒ Place pan over medium heat, bring to a simmer and mix with lemon juice.

⇒ Cook for 30 minutes, stirring all the time, take off heat and serve in small dessert bowls.

Nutrition: calories 258, fat 0,2, carbs 62,6, fiber 1,4, protein 0,9

100) Macaroons with Lemon Curd

Preparation Time: 10 minutes   **Cooking Time: 40 minutes**   **Servings:4**

Ingredients:

- 1 egg white
- 3 cups coconut flakes
- 2/3 cup almond milk
- ½ teaspoon vanilla extract
- 1 teaspoon lemon juice
- 1 teaspoon lemon zest

For the lemon curd:

- 5 tablespoons ghee, softened
- ½ cup raw honey
- 2 egg yolks
- 2 eggs
- 1 teaspoon lemon zest, grated
- 2/3 cup lemon juice

Directions:

⇒ In a bowl, mix honey with ghee and stir with a mixer for 3 minutes.

⇒ Add 2 egg yolks and 2 eggs and mix again well.

⇒ Add 2/3 cup lemon juice and mix 1 minute more.

⇒ Transfer this to a saucepan, heat up over medium-low heat and cook for 15 minutes stirring often.

⇒ Add 1 teaspoon lemon zest, stir, take off heat, transfer to a bowl and keep in the fridge for now.

⇒ In a bowl, mix coconut flakes with almond milk, 1 egg white, vanilla extract, 1 teaspoon lemon juice, 1 teaspoon lemon zest and stir well.

⇒ Shape small cookies, arrange them on a lined baking sheet, place in the oven at 325 degrees F and bake 20 minutes.

⇒ Take cookies out of the oven, leave aside for 5 minutes and arrange them on a platter.

⇒ Fill each macaroon with the lemon curd you've made and serve.

Nutrition: calories 638, fat 50, carbs 47, fiber 6,4, protein 8,2

101) Berry and Dates Cheesecake

Preparation Time: 2 hours and 10 minutes   **Cooking Time: 0 minutes**   **Servings:4**

Ingredients:

For the crust:

- ½ cup pecans
- ½ cup macadamia nuts
- ½ cup dates
- ½ cup walnuts

For the filling:

- 1 cup date paste

- 3 cups cashews, soaked for 3 hours
- ½ cup almond milk
- 2 cups strawberries
- ¾ cup coconut oil
- ¼ cup lime juice
- Sliced limes for serving
- Sliced strawberries for serving

Directions:

⇒ Put nuts, walnuts, dates and pecans in a food processor and blend well.

⇒ Put 3 spoons of crust mix each part of a muffin tin, press well and leave aside for now.

⇒ Put cashews, strawberries, date paste, lime juice, almond milk and coconut oil in the food processor and blend well.

⇒ Put 3 spoons of filling mix on top of crust mix, place in the freezer and keep for 2 hours.

⇒ Transfer cheesecakes on a platter, top with strawberries and limes and serve.

Nutrition: calories 1569, fat 130,6, fiber 15,4, carbs 99,9, protein 25,7

Chapter 10 -   Paleo Gillian's Meal Plan – for Women

Day 1

2) Almond Green Muffins | Calories 174

16) Rosemary Chicken Soup | Calories 459

32) Leeks Mix | Calories 222

43) Avocado Dip | Calories 316

51) Baked Turkey and Eggplant | Calories 362

64) Garlic Halibut Mix | Calories 1150

Total Calories 2683

Day 3

7) Coconut Bars | Calories 427

23) Sweet Potato and Carrot Soup | Calories 371

33) Root Veggie Stew | Calories 145

50) Sage Chicken and Turkey Mix | Calories 401

55) Chicken Balls and Sauce | Calories 552

75) Dill Trout | Calories 279

Total Calories 2175

Day 5

13) Avocado and Pumpkin Sandwich | Calories 310

19) Chili Carrot and Beet Soup | Calories 139

38) Maple Beets | Calories 141

45) Tahini Cauliflower Spread | Calories 183

58) Lamb and Squash Mix | Calories 775

83) Chicken and Berries Salad | Calories 916

Total Calories 2464

Day 7

8) Chicken and Veggie Rolls | Calories 274

25) Tomato and Beef Stew | Calories 412

41) Chives Cauliflower Bites | Calories 194

49) Stuffed Avocado | Calories 308

61) Beef with Asparagus and Mushrooms | Calories 284

87) Greens and Orange Salad | Calories 427

Total Calories 1899

Day 2

3) Lemony Pancakes | Calories 237

19) Chili Carrot and Beet Soup | Calories 139

35) Maple and Chili Asparagus | Calories 110

42) Lemon Cashew Spread | Calories 99

63) Cilantro Shrimp | Calories 218

77) Veggie and Eggs Salad | Calories 240

Total Calories 1043

Day 4

10) Coconut Zucchini and Leek Frittata | Calories 384

30) Root Veggie Stew | Calories 293

40) Cilantro Potatoes | Calories 220

48) Turkey Muffins | Calories 117

60) Beef and Basil Sauce | Calories 854

90) Tomato and Olives Salad | Calories 194

Total Calories 2062

Day 6

5) Spiced Waffles | Calories 225

28) Pumpkin and Chicken Stew | Calories 222

36) Garlic Coconut Squash | Calories 80

47) Cilantro Egg Bites | Calories 87

56) Slow Cooked Beef and Onions | Calories 1689

69) Citrus Calamari Mix | Calories 1108

Total Calories 3411

Chapter 11 - Conclusion

Always remember to consult with your medical professional before starting any dietary path.

I hope this book can be the springboard to start your long term transformation journey

You can check out (or give away) the other books in the series, just search for Kaylee Gillian.

Regards

Kaylee

Paleo Diet Cookbook for Men

Paleo Gillian's Meal Plan| Sculpt Your Body by Following a Carb-Free Eating Plan

By Kaylee Gillian

Chapter 1 -   Introduction

Paleo Diet is based on the idea that even modern men should eat as it was done in the distant past, this not only to ensure a healthy weight but also to keep healthy.

In order to stay healthy, according to Cordain, it is necessary to follow a diet very rich in animal proteins in which carbohydrates are completely excluded except those contained in fruits and vegetables. It is also important to associate to the paleolithic diet a regular physical activity: our ancestors in fact were not sedentary as they had to struggle every day to get the food they needed as they could not buy it easily in markets or supermarkets.

According to the creator, it would be a very simple diet to follow and always suitable, so not only in case you want to lose weight.

Have many small meals and not a few large ones; this also reduces hormonal (insulin) stimulation compared to that caused by larger, more concentrated meals.

Eat red or white meat (even if today's meat is treated compared to millions of years ago and loses many nutritional values compared to the paleolithic one; it is not a coincidence that farm animals are given feed with cereals inside, when they were free, however, they ate what nature had imposed) and carbohydrates taken from fruits and vegetables, avoiding pasta, bread, cookies, rusks, rice and all derivatives of cereals

Dissociate foods correctly, that is avoid mixing different proteins, in this way each food will be better digested and absorbed by the body.

Do physical activity: Paleolithic man went to hunt for food, he did not sit on a sofa watching TV, and made a fight to kill the animal; now instead we go to the supermarket and everything is already ready, so it is very important to do some sport.

With this diet, also associated with a zone diet, I was able to "bring back to the roots" many people in a short time, devastated by dietary regimes that unfortunately today's society imposes on us. Happy re-entry into today's civilization or happy beginning of a new era...paleo!

Chapter 2 -   Breakfast Recipes

1) *Turkey and Cranberry Sandwich*

Preparation Time: 5 minutes   **Cooking Time:**   **Servings:1**

Ingredients:

- 2 turkey breast slices, skinless, boneless and roasted
- 2 tablespoons walnuts, toasted and chopped
- 2 slices paleo coconut bread

- 2 tablespoons cranberry chutney
- ¼ cup baby arugula

Directions:

⇒ In a bowl, mix the walnuts with the chutney, stir and spread on one paleo slice of bread.

⇒ Add the turkey slices and the arugula, top with the other slice of bread and serve.

Nutrition: calories 347, fat 12,7, fiber 13,6, carbs 37,4, protein 28,6

2) *Coconut Berry Smoothie*

Preparation Time: 5 minutes   **Cooking Time:**   **Servings:2**

Ingredients:

- 2 cups blueberries
- 1 teaspoon lemon zest, grated
- ½ cup coconut milk

- 1 teaspoon cinnamon powder
- 3 cups water

Directions:

⇒ In a blender, combine all the ingredients, pulse well, divide into 2 glasses and serve for breakfast.

Nutrition: calories 222, fat 14,8, fiber 4,9, carbs 24,5, protein 2,5

3) *Lemon Kale Smoothie*

Preparation Time: 5 minutes   **Cooking Time:**   **Servings:2**

Ingredients:

- 1 small cucumber, peeled and chopped
- 1 green apple, chopped
- Juice of ½ lemon
- Juice of ½ lime

- 1 tablespoon ginger, finely grated
- 1 cup kale, chopped
- 1 cup coconut water

Directions:

⇒ In a blender, combine all the ingredients, pulse well, divide into 2 glasses and serve for breakfast.

Nutrition: calories 138, fat 1, fiber 5,8, carbs 32,1, protein 3,6

4) *Cabbage and Berry Smoothie*

Preparation Time: 5 minutes   **Cooking Time:**   **Servings:2**

Ingredients:

- 1 small red bell pepper, seeded and roughly chopped
- 5 strawberries, halved
- 1 tomato, cut into 4 wedges
- 1 cup red cabbage, chopped

- ½ cup raspberries
- 8 ounces water
- 2 ice cubes for serving

Directions:

⇒ In a blender, combine all the ingredients and pulse well. Divide into glasses and serve.   ⇒

Nutrition: calories 200, fat 5, fiber 11, carbs 20, protein 9

5) Mint Berry Smoothie

Preparation Time: 10 minutes   **Cooking Time:**   **Servings:2**

Ingredients:

- 1 and ½ cups kiwi, chopped
- 1 and ½ cups frozen strawberries, chopped
- 8 mint leaves

- 2 cups crushed ice
- ¼ cup water

Directions:

⇒ In a blender, combine all the ingredients and pulse well.
Divide into glasses and serve.

Nutrition: calories 59, fat 0,5, fiber 4,7, carbs 13,7, protein 1,9

6) Parsley Banana Smoothie

Preparation Time: 5 minutes   **Cooking Time:**   **Servings:6**

Ingredients:

- 1 bunch parsley, roughly chopped
- 1 small avocado, pitted and peeled
- 2 pears, peeled and chopped
- 1 green apple, chopped

- 6 bananas, peeled and roughly chopped
- 1 cup ice
- 1 cup water

Directions:

⇒ In a blender, combine all the ingredients and pulse well.
Divide into glasses and serve for breakfast.

Nutrition: calories 234, fat 1,5, fiber 8.4, carbs 45,7, protein 2,3

7) Coconut Smoothie

Preparation Time: 5 minutes   **Cooking Time:**   **Servings:2**

Ingredients:

- 1 cup ice
- 2 peaches, peeled and chopped

- 1 teaspoon lemon zest, grated
- 1 cup cold coconut milk

Directions:

⇒ In a blender, combine all the ingredients and pulse well.
Divide into glasses and serve.

Nutrition: calories 336, fat 29, fiber 5, carbs 20,9, protein 4,2

8) Walnut and Hemp Bowls

Preparation Time: 5 minutes   **Cooking Time: 50 minutes**   **Servings:6**

Ingredients:

- 2 teaspoons cinnamon powder
- 1 and ½ cups coconut flour
- 2 teaspoons nutmeg, ground
- ½ cup coconut flakes, unsweetened

- 2 teaspoons vanilla extract
- ½ cup walnuts, chopped
- 1/3 cup coconut oil, melted
- ¼ cup hemp hearts

Directions:

⇒ Spread all the ingredients out onto a lined baking sheet, toss to combine, and bake at 300 degrees F for 50 minutes, stirring every 10 minutes.

⇒ Divide into bowls and serve for breakfast.

Nutrition: calories 403, fat 28,6, fiber 17,4, carbs 28,5, protein 10,9

9) Almond Berry Bowls

Preparation Time: 5 minutes   **Cooking Time: 0 minutes**   Servings:2

Ingredients:

- 2 tablespoons pumpkin seeds
- 2 tablespoons almonds, chopped
- 1 tablespoon chia seeds

- A handful blueberries
- 1 cup almond milk

Directions:

⇒ Divide the almond milk into 2 bowls, then divide the seeds, almonds and blueberries, toss to combine and serve.

Nutrition: calories 400, fat 37,1, fiber 6,2, carbs 16,4, protein 7,2

10) Coconut Orange Bowls

Preparation Time: 5 minutes   **Cooking Time: 0 minutes**   Servings:2

Ingredients:

- 2 cups coconut milk
- ½ cup chia seeds
- Juice of ¼ lemon

- Zest from 1 orange, grated
- 1 tablespoon vanilla extract

Directions:

⇒ In a large bowl, combine all the ingredients and toss.   ⇒ Divide into 2 bowls and serve.

Nutrition: calories 672, fat 61,8, fiber 10,3, carbs 27,4, protein 8

11) Maple Coconut Bowls

Preparation Time: 10 minutes   **Cooking Time: 35 minutes**   Servings:4

Ingredients:

- 3 cups coconut flakes, unsweetened
- 1 and ½ cups almonds, chopped
- ½ cup sesame seeds
- ½ cup sunflower seeds

- ½ teaspoon cinnamon powder
- 2 tablespoons chia seeds
- 1 teaspoon vanilla extract
- 2 tablespoons coconut oil, melted

Directions:

⇒ In a bowl, mix almonds with sunflower seeds, sesame seeds, coconut, chia seeds and the cinnamon and stir.

⇒ Heat up a pot over medium heat, add the oil, vanilla and whisk, cook for about 1 minute and pour over the seeds and coconut mixture.

⇒ Stir everything, spread on a lined baking sheet, bake at 300 degrees F for 25 minutes, stirring the mixture after 15 minutes.

⇒ Divide the granola into bowls and serve.

Nutrition: calories 615, fat 47,1, fiber 10,8, carbs 45, protein 9,8

12) Beef and Chili Rolls

Preparation Time: 10 minutes   **Cooking Time: 15 minutes**   **Servings:2**

Ingredients:

- 0,5 oz green chilies, chopped
- 1 small yellow onion, chopped
- 4 eggs, egg yolks and whites separated
- ¼ cup cilantro, chopped
- 1 red bell pepper, finely cut into strips

- 2 tomatoes, chopped
- ½ cup beef meat, ground and browned for 10 minutes
- 1 avocado, peeled, pitted and chopped
- A drizzle of olive oil

Directions:

⇒ Heat up a pan with some olive oil over medium-high heat, add half of the egg whites after you've whisked them in a bowl, spread evenly, cook for 1 minute on each side and transfer to a plate.

⇒ Repeat the process with the rest of the egg whites and leave the egg "burritos" to one side.

⇒ Heat up the same pan over medium-high heat, add the onions, stir and sauté for 2 minutes.

⇒ Add chilies, bell pepper, tomato, meat, and cilantro, stir and cook for 5 minutes.

⇒ Add egg yolks, stir well and cook everything for 4-5 minutes more.

⇒ Divide the egg white burritos between 2 plates, divide the meat mixture, also divide the avocado, roll and serve for breakfast.

Nutrition: calories 489, fat 37,4, fiber 9,8, carbs 22,2, protein 21,3

13) Poached Eggs with Artichokes and Lemon Sauce

Preparation Time: 20 minutes   **Cooking Time: 30 minutes**   **Servings:2**

Ingredients:

- 1 egg white, whisked
- 4 eggs
- ¾ cup balsamic vinegar
- 4 ounces shallots, cooked and chopped
- 4 artichoke hearts, chopped
- A pinch of sea salt and black pepper

For the sauce:

- 1 tablespoon lemon juice
- ¾ cup ghee, softened
- 4 egg yolks
- ¼ teaspoon sweet paprika

Directions:

⇒ Put artichoke hearts in a bowl, add the vinegar, toss well to combine and leave aside for 20 minutes

⇒ In a bowl, mix the egg yolks with paprika and lemon juice and whisk.

⇒ Put some water into a saucepan and bring to a simmer over medium heat.

⇒ Put the bowl with the egg yolks over the simmering water and stir constantly.

⇒ Add melted ghee gradually, stir until the sauce thickens and take off heat.

⇒ Drain artichokes, arrange them on a lined baking sheet, brush them with the egg white, sprinkle salt, pepper and the chopped shallots on top, and bake at 375 degrees F for 20 minutes.

⇒ Heat up a saucepan with some water, bring to a simmer over medium heat, crack the 4 whole eggs into the pan, poach them for 1 minute and divide them between plates.

⇒ Add the baked artichokes on the side, drizzle the egg yolk sauce all over and serve.

Nutrition: calories 1130, fat 94,9, fiber 17,6, carbs 46,7, protein 30,6

14) Tomato and Kale Scramble

Preparation Time: 10 minutes   **Cooking Time: 10 minutes**   Servings:1

Ingredients:

- 2 eggs, whisked
- ¼ teaspoon rosemary, dried
- ½ cup cherry tomatoes halved
- 1 and ½ cups kale, chopped

- ½ teaspoon coconut oil, melted
- 3 tablespoons water
- 1 teaspoon balsamic vinegar
- ¼ avocado, peeled, pitted and chopped

Directions:

⇒ Heat up a pan with the oil over medium heat, add the water, kale, rosemary, and tomatoes, stir, cover and cook for 5 minutes.

⇒ Add the eggs, stir and scramble everything for 4 minutes more.

⇒ Add the vinegar, toss, transfer this to a plate, top with chopped avocado and serve.

Nutrition: calories 403, fat 21,3, fiber 15,5, carbs 26,2, protein 24

15) Scallion Muffins

Preparation Time: 10 minutes   **Cooking Time: 15 minutes**   Servings:4

Ingredients:

- 4 eggs
- 10 ham slices
- 4 tablespoons scallions, chopped

- A pinch of black pepper
- ½ teaspoon sweet paprika
- 1 tablespoon melted ghee

Directions:

⇒ Grease a muffin pan with the melted ghee and divide the ham slices in each muffin mold to shape your cups.

⇒ In a bowl, mix the eggs with scallions, pepper, and paprika, whisk well, divide this into the ham cups, and bake at 400 degrees F for 15 minutes.

⇒ Divide between plates and serve for breakfast.

Nutrition: calories 214, fat 14,2, fiber 1,2, carbs 3,6, protein 17,3

Chapter 3 -   Soup & Stew Recipes

16) Herbed Chicken and Olives Stew

Preparation Time: 15 minutes   **Cooking Time: 2 hours**   **Servings:4**

Ingredients:

- 10 garlic cloves, peeled
- 30 black olives, pitted
- 2 pounds chicken breasts, skinless, boneless and cubed
- 2 cups chicken stock
- 25 ounces tomatoes, peeled, chopped

- 2 tablespoon rosemary, chopped
- 2 tablespoons parsley, chopped
- 2 tablespoons basil, chopped
- A pinch of sea salt and black pepper
- A drizzle of extra virgin olive oil

Directions:

⇒ Heat up a large saucepan with a drizzle of olive oil over medium-high heat, add the chicken, salt and pepper, and cook for 4 minutes.

⇒ Add garlic, stir and brown for 2 minutes more.

⇒ Add chicken stock, tomatoes, olives, thyme, and rosemary, stir, cover saucepan and bake in the oven at 325 degrees F for 1 hour.

⇒ Add parsley and basil, stir, bake for 45 more minutes, divide into bowls and serve.

Nutrition: calories 553, fat 24,8, fiber 4,1, carbs 13, protein 68,5

17) Leeks Oxtail and Tomato Stew

Preparation Time: 15 minutes   **Cooking Time: 6 hours**   **Servings:8**

Ingredients:

- 4 and ½ pounds oxtail, cut into medium chunks
- 2 tablespoons extra virgin olive oil
- 2 leeks, chopped
- 4 carrots, chopped
- 2 celery sticks, chopped
- 4 thyme springs, chopped
- 4 rosemary springs, chopped

- 4 cloves
- 4 bay leaves
- Black pepper to taste
- 2 tablespoons coconut flour
- 25 ounces plum tomatoes, peeled, chopped
- 1-quart beef stock

Directions:

⇒ In a roasting pan, mix oxtail with black pepper and half of the oil, toss and bake at 425 degrees F for 20 minutes.

⇒ Heat up a large saucepan with the rest of the oil over medium heat, add leeks, celery, and carrots, stir and cook for 4 minutes.

⇒ Add thyme, rosemary and bay leaves, stir and cook everything for 20 minutes.

⇒ Add flour and cloves to veggies and stir.

⇒ Also add tomatoes, the oxtail, its cooking juices and stock, stir, increase heat to high, bring to a boil, place the pot in the oven and bake at 325 degrees F for 5 hours.

⇒ Take the oxtail out of the pot, discard bones, return it to the pot, toss, divide the stew into bowls and serve.

Nutrition: calories 580, fat 32,6, fiber 3,1, carbs 12,8, protein 59,7

18) Cayenne Tomato and Eggplant Stew

Preparation Time: 10 minutes   **Cooking Time: 30 minutes**   **Servings:3**

Ingredients:

- 1 eggplant, chopped
- 1 yellow onion, chopped
- 2 tomatoes, chopped
- 1 teaspoon cumin powder

- A pinch of sea salt and black pepper
- 1 cup tomato puree
- A pinch of cayenne pepper
- ½ cup water

Directions:

⇒ Heat up a saucepan over medium-high heat, add the water, tomato paste, salt, pepper, cayenne and cumin and stir well.

⇒ Add the eggplant, tomato, and onion, stir, bring to a boil, reduce heat to medium, cook for 30 minutes, divide into bowls and serve.

Nutrition: calories 102, fat 0,8, fiber 8,8, carbs 23,4, protein 4,1

19) Nutmeg Coconut and Squash Cream

Preparation Time: 10 minutes   **Cooking Time: 50 minutes**   **Servings:4**

Ingredients:

- 1 butternut squash, halved lengthwise and deseeded
- 14 ounces coconut milk
- A pinch of sea salt and black pepper
- A handful parsley, chopped
- A pinch of nutmeg, ground

Directions:

⇒ Arrange the butternut squash halves on a lined baking sheet, place in the oven at 350 degrees F, bake for 45 minutes, cool down, scoop the flesh and transfer it to a large saucepan.

⇒ Add half of the coconut milk, blend using an immersion blender and then heat everything up over medium-low heat.

⇒ Add the rest of the coconut milk, salt, black pepper, nutmeg and parsley, blend using your immersion blender for a few seconds, cook for about 4 minutes, ladle into bowls and serve.

Nutrition: calories 245, fat 23,7, fiber 3, carbs 9,8, protein 2,7

20) Lemon Broccoli and Pesto Soup

Preparation Time: 10 minutes   **Cooking Time: 20 minutes**   **Servings:4**

Ingredients:

- 1 yellow onion, chopped
- 2 tablespoons olive oil
- 1 celery stick, chopped
- Zest of ½ lemon, grated
- 1-quart veggie stock
- 17 ounces water
- 1 teaspoon cumin, ground
- 1 broccoli head, florets separated
- 3 garlic cloves, minced
- 2 bay leaves
- Juice of ½ lemon
- A pinch of sea salt and black pepper

  For the pesto:
- ½ cup almonds, chopped
- 1 garlic clove
- 2 tablespoons lemon juice
- 2 tablespoons olive oil
- 4 tablespoons green olives, pitted and chopped

Directions:

⇒ Heat up a large saucepan with 2 tablespoons olive oil over medium-high heat, add onion, lemon zest and a pinch of salt, stir and cook for 3 minutes.

⇒ Add celery and 3 garlic cloves, stir and cook for 1 minute more.

⇒ Add stock, cumin, water, and black pepper, stir, cover, bring to a boil and simmer for 10 minutes.

⇒ Add bay leaves and broccoli, stir, cover again and cook for 6 minutes more.

⇒ Take soup off the heat, discard bay leaves, transfer to a blender and pulse well. Add juice from ½ lemon, pulse again, return to the pot and heat up again over medium-low heat.

⇒ Meanwhile, in a food processor, blend the almonds with 1 garlic clove, 2 tablespoon lemon juice, 2 tablespoons olive oil and the green olives. Ladle the soup into bowls, top with the pesto you've just made and serve hot.

Nutrition: calories 201, fat 16,8, fiber 4,8, carbs 14,6, protein 5,4

21) Tomato and Peppers Soup

Preparation Time: 10 minutes   **Cooking Time: 0 minutes**   **Servings:4**

Ingredients:

- 8 tomatoes
- 1 red onion, chopped
- 1 cucumber, peeled and chopped
- 1 red bell pepper, chopped
- 1 green bell pepper, chopped
- 1 red chili pepper, chopped
- 3 garlic cloves

- 1 cup tomato juice
- 1 cup water
- 2 tablespoon apple cider vinegar
- Zest of ½ orange, grated
- ¾ cup olive oil
- A pinch of sea salt and black pepper

Directions:

⇒ In a blender, combine all the ingredients and pulse them well.

⇒ Divide the gazpacho into bowls and serve it cold.

Nutrition: calories 417, fat 38,5, fiber 5,2, carbs 21, protein 3,9

22) Mushrooms and Kale Soup

Preparation Time: 10 minutes   **Cooking Time: 15 minutes**   **Servings:4**

Ingredients:

- 1 yellow onion, chopped
- 2 carrots, chopped
- 6 mushrooms, chopped
- 1 red chili pepper, chopped
- 2 celery sticks, chopped
- 1 tablespoon coconut oil
- A pinch of sea salt and black pepper

- 4 garlic cloves, minced
- 4 ounces kale, chopped
- 15 oz fresh tomatoes, peeled, chopped
- 1 zucchini, chopped
- 1-quart veggie stock
- 1 bay leaf
- A handful parsley, chopped for serving

Directions:

⇒ Set your instant pot on Sauté mode, add oil and heat it up.

⇒ Add celery, carrots, onion, a pinch of salt and black pepper, stir and cook for 2 minutes.

⇒ Add chili pepper, garlic and the mushrooms, stir and cook for 2 minutes.

⇒ Add tomatoes, stock, bay leaf, kale and zucchinis, stir, cover pot and cook on High for 10 minutes.

⇒ Release pressure, stir soup again, discard the bay leaf, ladle into bowls, sprinkle the parsley on top and serve.

Nutrition: calories 109, fat 3,9, fiber 4,3, carbs 16,9, protein 4,1

23) Chicken, Tomato and Kale Soup

Preparation Time: 10 minutes   **Cooking Time: 15 minutes**   **Servings:2**

Ingredients:

- 1 red bell pepper, chopped
- 1 teaspoon coconut oil
- 1 yellow onion, chopped
- ¼ cup jalapeno peppers, chopped
- 2 garlic cloves, minced
- 1 tablespoon ghee, melted
- 1 teaspoon cumin, ground
- 1 teaspoon coriander, ground
- 1 teaspoon oregano, dried
- 1 and ½ cups chicken breast, skinless, boneless, cooked and shredded
- 2 and ½ cups chicken stock

- 2 cups kale, torn
- Zest of 1 lime, grated
- Juice of 1 lime
- A pinch of sea salt and black pepper
- 15 ounces fresh tomatoes, peeled, chopped
- 2 tablespoons spring onions, chopped
- 3 tablespoons pumpkin seeds, toasted
- 1 avocado, peeled, pitted and sliced
- 1 teaspoon sweet paprika
- 3 tablespoons coriander, chopped

Directions:

⇒ Heat up a large saucepan with the oil over medium heat, add the onion, stir and sauté for 2 minutes.

⇒ Add red bell peppers, the garlic, jalapenos, oregano, cumin, coriander, and ghee, stir and cook for 1 minute more.

⇒ Add tomatoes, kale, chicken, lime zest, stock, lime juice, salt and pepper, stir, bring to a boil, cook for 5 minutes and take off the heat.

⇒ Ladle the soup into bowls, top with pumpkin seeds, green onion, paprika, chopped coriander and avocado and serve.

Nutrition: calories 1227, fat 53,2, fiber 14,2, carbs 60,7, protein 127,6

24) Broccoli and Spinach Soup

Preparation Time: 10 minutes   **Cooking Time: 25 minutes**   **Servings:6**

Ingredients:

- 2 leeks, chopped
- 2 tablespoons ghee
- 4 celery sticks, chopped
- 4 garlic cloves, minced
- 2 broccoli heads, florets separated
- 1 small cauliflower head, florets separated

- 2 handfuls spinach, chopped
- 8 cups veggie stock
- 1 handful parsley, chopped
- 1 tablespoon coconut cream
- A pinch of nutmeg, ground
- Black pepper to taste

Directions:

⇒ Heat up a large saucepan with the ghee over medium heat, add garlic and leeks, stir and cook for 3 minutes.

⇒ Add the broccoli, celery and cauliflower, stir and cook for 5 minutes,

⇒ Add stock, bring to a boil, cover saucepan and cook for 15 minutes.

⇒ Add parsley, spinach, black pepper and the nutmeg, stir and blend using an immersion blender.

⇒ Ladle soup into bowls and serve with the coconut cream on top.

Nutrition: calories 120, fat 8, fiber 4,4, carbs 16, protein 4

25) Mustard Mushroom Cream

Preparation Time: 10 minutes   **Cooking Time: 20 minutes**   **Servings:4**

Ingredients:

- 1 ounce dried porcini mushrooms
- 1 leek, chopped
- 2 tablespoons olive oil
- 1 celery stick, chopped
- 3 garlic cloves, chopped
- 14 brown mushrooms, chopped
- 1 tablespoon thyme, chopped
- 3 cups veggie stock

- 1 sweet potato, peeled and chopped
- 2 bay leaves
- ½ teaspoon Dijon mustard
- 1 teaspoon lemon zest, grated
- ½ teaspoon black pepper
- 1 tablespoon lemon juice
- 3 tablespoons coconut butter

Directions:

⇒ Put dried mushrooms in a bowl, cover them with boiling water, leave aside for 10 minutes, strain, reserve water and chop them.

⇒ Heat up a large saucepan with the oil over medium heat, add celery and leek, stir and cook for 5 minutes.

⇒ Add mushrooms, thyme, garlic and sweet potatoes, stir and cook for 1 minute.

⇒ Add dried mushrooms and half of their liquid, stock, bay leaves, mustard, black pepper and lemon zest, stir, cover pan and simmer soup over medium heat for 15 minutes.

⇒ Discard bay leaves, use an immersion blender to make your mushroom cream, add lemon juice and the coconut butter, stir well, ladle into bowls and serve.

Nutrition: calories 171, fat 8,8, fiber 4,2, carbs 18,9, protein 4,8

26) Garlic Cod Soup

Preparation Time: 2 hours and 10 minutes   **Cooking Time: 30 minutes**   **Servings:4**

Ingredients:

- 1 pound cod fillets, skinless, boneless and cubed
- 10 garlic cloves, minced
- 3 tablespoons olive oil
- 1 tablespoon lemon juice
- ¼ cup parsley, chopped
- 1 yellow onion, chopped
- 2 tomatoes, chopped

- 1 tablespoon tomato paste
- 2 bay leaves
- 2 and ½ cups water
- A pinch of sea salt and black pepper
- 1 pound shrimp, peeled and deveined
- 10 cherry tomatoes, halved
- 1 pound mussels, scrubbed

Directions:

⇒ In a bowl, mix 6 garlic cloves with 2 tablespoons oil, parsley, lemon juice and the fish, toss, cover the bowl and keep in the fridge for 2 hours.

⇒ Heat up a large saucepan with the rest of the oil over medium-high heat, add the onion, stir and cook for 2 minutes.

⇒ Add the rest of the garlic, the tomatoes, tomato paste, bay leaves, water, salt, pepper and the fish, stir, bring to a simmer and cook for 10 minutes.

⇒ Add shrimp, cherry tomatoes and mussels, stir, cook for 6 minutes more, ladle into bowls and serve.

Nutrition: calories 508, fat 17, fiber 2,3, carbs 16, protein 71,1

27) Coconut Shrimp Soup

Preparation Time: 10 minutes   **Cooking Time: 30 minutes**   **Servings:4**

Ingredients:

- 5 tablespoons curry paste
- 1 tablespoon coconut oil, melted
- 1 big chicken breast, skinless, boneless and cut into thin strips
- 4 tablespoons coconut aminos
- 2 cups chicken stock
- Juice of 1 lime
- 1 and ½ cups coconut milk
- 1 pound shrimp, peeled and deveined

- ½ cup coconut cream
- A small broccoli head, florets separated
- 5 Chinese broccoli leaves, chopped
- 1 zucchini, chopped
- 1 carrot, chopped
- 1 cucumber, chopped
- 1 tablespoon cilantro, chopped for serving

Directions:

⇒ Heat up a large saucepan with the oil over medium heat, add curry paste, stir and heat up for 1 minute.

⇒ Add the chicken, stir and cook for 1 minute more.

⇒ Add stock and lime juice, stir and cook for 2 minutes.

⇒ Add coconut cream, aminos and coconut milk, stir and cook for 10 minutes.

⇒ Add broccoli leaves, broccoli florets and carrots, stir and cook for 3 minutes.

⇒ Add shrimp and zucchini, stir and cook for 2 minutes.

⇒ Ladle into bowls, top with cilantro and cucumber and serve.

Nutrition: calories 1252, fat 98,5, fiber 11,2, carbs 40,8, protein 62,3

28) Coconut Zucchini Cream

Preparation Time: 10 minutes   **Cooking Time: 20 minutes**   **Servings:4**

Ingredients:

- 1 onion, chopped
- 3 zucchinis, cut into medium chunks
- 2 tablespoons coconut milk
- 2 garlic cloves, minced

- 4 cups chicken stock
- 2 tablespoons coconut oil
- A pinch of sea salt and black pepper

Directions:

⇒ Heat up a large saucepan with the oil over medium heat, add zucchinis, garlic, and onion, stir and cook for 5 minutes.

⇒ Add stock, salt, pepper, stir, bring to a boil, cover pan, simmer soup for 20 minutes and take off heat.

⇒ Add coconut milk, blend using an immersion blender, ladle into bowls and serve.

Nutrition: calories 122, fat 9,5, fiber 2,4, carbs 9,1, protein 3

29) Curry Coconut Soup

Preparation Time: 10 minutes   **Cooking Time: 15 minutes**   **Servings:2**

Ingredients:

- 1 brown onion, chopped
- 1 tablespoon coconut oil
- 2 zucchinis, cubed
- A pinch of sea salt and black pepper
- 2 teaspoons turmeric powder
- 3 garlic cloves, chopped

- 1 teaspoon curry powder
- 1 cup coconut milk
- 1 cup veggie stock
- 2 tablespoons lime juice
- 1 tablespoon cilantro, chopped

Directions:

⇒ Heat up a large saucepan with the oil over medium heat, add onion, stir and sauté for 4 minutes.

⇒ Add garlic, salt, pepper, and zucchinis, stir and cook for 1 minute.

⇒ Add turmeric and curry powder, stir well and cook for 1 minute more.

⇒ Add coconut milk and stock, stir, bring to a boil, cover pan and simmer soup for 10 minutes.

⇒ Add lime juice and cilantro, stir, ladle into bowls and serve.

Nutrition: calories 414, fat 32,4, fiber 6,9, carbs 23,8, protein 6,4

30) Shallot and Cauliflower Cream

Preparation Time: 10 minutes   **Cooking Time: 20 minutes**   **Servings:2**

Ingredients:

- 1 yellow onion, chopped
- 2 tablespoons olive oil
- 1 cauliflower head, florets separated and chopped
- 3 cups veggie stock
- 3 garlic cloves, minced

- A pinch of sea salt and black pepper
- ¾ cup shallots, cooked and chopped
- 1 teaspoon coconut oil, melted
- 1 egg
- 2 tablespoons cilantro, chopped

Directions:

⇒ Heat up a large saucepan with the olive oil over medium heat, add the onion, stir and sauté for 4 minutes.

⇒ Add stock, cauliflower and garlic, stir, bring to a boil, reduce heat to medium-low, season with salt and black pepper, cover the saucepan and simmer soup for 10 minutes.

⇒ Meanwhile, put water in a pot, bring to a boil, place a bowl on top of boiling water, crack the egg into the bowl, whisk it for 3 minutes and take off the heat.

⇒ Blend the soup using an immersion blender, add whisked egg and blend again.

⇒ Ladle into bowls, sprinkle crumbled shallots and cilantro on top and serve.

Nutrition: calories 291, fat 21,7, fiber 4,6, carbs 26,9, protein 7,8

31) Sweet Potato and Nettle Cream

Preparation Time: 10 minutes **Cooking Time: 20 minutes** **Servings:3**

Ingredients:

- 1 tablespoon coconut oil, melted
- 1 cup sweet potato, chopped
- 1 yellow onion, chopped
- ½ broccoli head, florets separated
- ½ cauliflower head, florets separated
- 3 garlic cloves, minced
- Zest of 1 lemon, grated
- 1 teaspoon Dijon mustard

- 3 and ½ cups veggie stock
- A pinch of sea salt and black pepper
- 4 cups nettles
- Juice of 1 lemon
- 5 thyme springs, leaves separated
- 2 small shallots, cooked and crumbled
- ½ cup coconut cream

Directions:

⇒ Heat up a large saucepan with the coconut oil over medium heat, add sweet potato, onion, broccoli, and cauliflower, stir and cook for 6 minutes.

⇒ Add the garlic, veggie stock, lemon zest, salt, pepper, and mustard, stir, bring to a boil, reduce the heat and simmer the soup for 10 minutes

⇒ Meanwhile, put some water in a pot, bring to a boil, cut nettles leaves with scissors, add the leaves to the boiling water, cook them for 2 minutes, drain and transfer them to the saucepan with the soup.

⇒ Cook for 3 minutes more, add lemon juice, blend everything using an immersion blender and then heat up the soup again.

⇒ Add thyme and coconut cream, stir, cook for 1 minute and ladle into soup bowls.

⇒ Top with the shallots and serve.

Nutrition: calories 766, fat 44,7, fiber 25,1, carbs 90,7, protein 16,1

32) Garlic Potato and Pine Nuts Cream

Preparation Time: 10 minutes **Cooking Time: 20 minutes** **Servings:2**

Ingredients:

- 4 tablespoons olive oil
- 5 garlic cloves, minced
- 1 sweet potato, chopped
- ½ teaspoon cumin seeds

- 14 ounces veggie stock
- A pinch of sea salt and black pepper
- 4 tablespoons pine nuts, toasted

Directions:

⇒ Heat up a large saucepan with the oil over medium heat, add the garlic, stir and cook for 4 minutes.

⇒ Add the sweet potato, stock, cumin, salt and black pepper, stir, bring to a boil and cook for 15 minutes.

⇒ Blend the soup using an immersion blender and mix with half of the pine nuts.

⇒ Blend again, ladle into bowls and sprinkle the rest of the pine nuts on top.

Nutrition: calories 445, fat 45, fiber 2,8, carbs 21,8, protein 4,1

Chapter 4 - Side Recipes

33) Asparagus and Green Onions Mix

Preparation Time: 10 minutes   **Cooking Time: 10 minutes**   **Servings:4**

Ingredients:

- 1 pound asparagus, trimmed
- A pinch of sea salt and black pepper
- 8 green onions, thinly sliced
- 2 tablespoons coconut oil

- 2 tablespoons balsamic vinegar
- 2 tablespoons walnuts, chopped
- 1 pound mushrooms, chopped

Directions:

⇒ In a bowl, mix the vinegar with salt, pepper and half of the oil and whisk.

⇒ Put some water in a large saucepan, bring to a boil over medium heat, add asparagus, cook for 3 minutes, drain and transfer to a bowl filled with cold water.

⇒ Heat up a pan with the rest of the oil over medium-high heat, add mushrooms and cook them for 4-5 minutes stirring from time to time.

⇒ Add onions, stir and cook for 1 minute.

⇒ Add drained asparagus, stir, cook 3 more minutes and take off heat.

⇒ Add vinegar mix, stir and divide between plates.

⇒ Sprinkle the walnuts at the end and serve as a side dish!

Nutrition: calories 141, fat 9,6, fiber 4,6, carbs 10,8, protein 7,5

34) Baked Mushrooms

Preparation Time: 10 minutes   **Cooking Time: 25 minutes**   **Servings:4**

Ingredients:

- 4 garlic cloves, minced
- 2 tablespoons extra virgin olive oil

- 16 ounces mushrooms, sliced
- A pinch of sea salt and black pepper

Directions:

⇒ In a baking dish, combine all the ingredients, toss, and bake at 375 degrees F for 25 minutes.

⇒ Divide everything between plates and serve as a side dish.

Nutrition: calories 89, fat 7,3, fiber 1,2, carbs 4,7, protein 3,8

35) Garlic and Basil Tomatoes

Preparation Time: 5 minutes   **Cooking Time: 20 minutes**   **Servings:4**

Ingredients:

- 2 tablespoons extra virgin olive oil
- 20 ounces colored cherry tomatoes, halved
- 6 garlic cloves, finely minced

- A pinch of sea salt and black pepper
- 1 tablespoon basil leaves, finely chopped

Directions:

⇒ In a baking dish, combine all the ingredients, place in the oven at 375 degrees F and bake for 20 minutes.

⇒ Divide between plates and serve as a side dish.

Nutrition: calories 91, fat 7,4, fiber 1,9, carbs 6,8, protein 2,1

36) Garlic Spinach

Preparation Time: 10 minutes   **Cooking Time: 33 minutes**   **Servings:3**

Ingredients:

- 3 cups spinach, torn
- 3 yellow onions, sliced
- 3 garlic cloves, finely minced
- A pinch of sea salt and black pepper
- 10 mushrooms, sliced
- 1 tablespoon coconut oil, melted
- 1 tablespoon balsamic vinegar
- 1 tablespoon ghee

Directions:

⇒ Heat up a pan with the oil and ghee over medium-high heat, add garlic and onions, stir and cook for 10 minutes.

⇒ Reduce temperature to low and cook onions for 20 minutes, stirring from time to time.

⇒ Add vinegar, mushrooms, salt and pepper, stir and cook for 10 minutes.

⇒ Add spinach, stir, cook for 3 minutes more, take off heat, divide between plates and serve as a side dish.

Nutrition: calories 146, fat 9,2, fiber 3,7, carbs 14,4, protein 4,2

37) Parsley Carrot Mash

Preparation Time: 6 minutes   **Cooking Time: 20 minutes**   **Servings:4**

Ingredients:

- 1 pound rutabaga, peeled and chopped
- A pinch of sea salt and black pepper
- 4 tablespoons ghee
- 1 pound carrots, chopped
- 1 tablespoon parsley, chopped

Directions:

⇒ Put rutabaga and carrots in a pot, add water to cover, place on stove, bring to a boil over medium heat and cook for 20 minutes.

⇒ Drain carrots and rutabaga, transfer them to a bowl, mash with a potato masher, mix with ghee, salt and pepper, stir well, divide between plates, sprinkle parsley on top and serve as a side dish.

Nutrition: calories 200, fat 13, fiber 5,7, carbs 12,4, protein 2,4

38) Balsamic Peppers and Capers Mix

Preparation Time: 10 minutes   **Cooking Time: 1 hour**   **Servings:4**

Ingredients:

- 6 bell peppers (green, yellow and red)
- 1 garlic clove, finely minced
- 2 tablespoon capers
- 2 tablespoons extra virgin olive oil
- ¼ cup balsamic vinegar
- A pinch of sea salt and black pepper
- 2 tablespoons parsley, finely chopped

Directions:

⇒ Arrange bell peppers on a lined baking sheet, place them in the oven at 400 degrees F and bake for 40 minutes.

⇒ Transfer bell peppers to a bowl, cover and leave them aside for 10 minutes.

⇒ Peel the peppers, discard seeds, cut into strips and transfer them to a bowl.

⇒ Add sea salt and pepper, vinegar, oil, garlic, capers and parsley, toss to coat, divide between plates and serve as a side dish.

Nutrition: calories 123, fat 7,5, fiber 2,6, carbs 14,2, protein 2

39) Herbed Potatoes

Preparation Time: 10 minutes   **Cooking Time: 25 minutes**   **Servings:3**

Ingredients:

- 2 pounds sweet potatoes, cut into wedges
- A pinch of sea salt and black pepper
- ¼ cup ghee, melted
- 3 teaspoons thyme and rosemary, dried

Directions:

⇒ In a bowl, mix potato wedges with ghee, salt, pepper and dried herbs and toss to coat.

⇒ Spread potatoes on a lined baking sheet and bake in the oven at 425 degrees F for 25 minutes.

⇒ Divide between plates and serve as a side dish.

Nutrition: calories 512, fat 7,7, fiber 13,1, carbs 85,6, protein 4,9

40) Lemon Chili Cabbage

Preparation Time: 10 minutes   **Cooking Time: 30 minutes**   **Servings:4**

Ingredients:

- 1 green cabbage head, cut into medium wedges
- A pinch of sea salt and black pepper
- A pinch of red chili flakes
- A pinch of garlic powder
- 2 tablespoons extra virgin olive oil
- Juice of 2 lemons

Directions:

⇒ Brush the cabbage with olive oil, salt and pepper, sprinkle garlic powder and pepper flakes, arrange it on a lined baking sheet and bake at 450 degrees F for 30 minutes, flipping the cabbage wedges halfway.

⇒ Divide between plates, drizzle the lemon juice on top and serve.

Nutrition: calories 118, fat 7,3, fiber 4,8, carbs 14, protein 2,7

41) Paprika Okra Mix

Preparation Time: 10 minutes   **Cooking Time: 25 minutes**   **Servings:3**

Ingredients:

- 18 okra pods, sliced
- A pinch of sea salt and black pepper
- 1 teaspoon sweet paprika
- 1 tablespoon extra-virgin olive oil

Directions:

⇒ Combine all the ingredients in a baking dish, place in the oven and bake at 425 degrees F for 15 minutes.

⇒ Divide between plates and serve as a side dish.

Nutrition: calories 107, fat 5, fiber 5,3, carbs 12,4, protein 3,2

Chapter 5 -   Snack & Appetizer Recipes

42) Hot Artichoke Bowls

Preparation Time: 10 minutes   **Cooking Time: 0 minutes**   **Servings:4**

Ingredients:

- 1 big romaine lettuce head, chopped
- ½ cup artichoke hearts, chopped
- ½ cup hot peppers, chopped
- ½ cup black olives, pitted and chopped
- For the dressing:
- 1 tablespoon parsley, chopped

- 1 garlic clove, minced
- 1 teaspoon oregano, dried
- Black pepper to taste
- A pinch of sea salt
- ¾ cup avocado oil
- ¼ cup red wine vinegar

Directions:

⇒ In a bowl, combine all the ingredients, toss, divide into small cups and serve as an appetizer.

Nutrition: calories 109, fat 7,2, fiber 5, carbs 10,2, protein 3

43) Banana and Walnut Snack

Preparation Time: 5 minutes   **Cooking Time: 1 hour and 30 minutes**   **Servings:6**

Ingredients:

- 2 and ¼ cup walnuts, chopped
- 1/3 cup coconut sugar
- 5 tablespoons coconut oil

- 1 cup coconut flakes, unsweetened
- 1 teaspoon vanilla extract
- 2 cups banana slices, dried

Directions:

⇒ In a crock pot, combine all the ingredients, cover and cook on Low for 1 hour and 30 minutes.

⇒ Divide everything into bowls and serve as a snack.

Nutrition: calories 464, fat 29, fiber 7,8, carbs 56,5, protein 5,3

44) Squash Wraps

Preparation Time: 10 minutes   **Cooking Time: 40 minutes**   **Servings:4**

Ingredients:

- 10 ounces turkey meat, cooked, sliced
- 2 pounds butternut squash, cubed
- 1 teaspoon chili powder

- 1 teaspoon garlic powder
- 1 teaspoon sweet paprika
- Black pepper to taste

Directions:

⇒ In a bowl, mix butternut squash cubes with chili powder, black pepper, garlic powder and paprika and toss to coat.

⇒ Wrap squash pieces in turkey slices, place them all on a lined baking sheet, place in the oven at 350 degrees F, bake for 20 minutes, flip and bake for 20 minutes more.

⇒ Arrange squash bites on a platter and serve.

Nutrition: calories 223, fat 3,8, fiber 4,5, carbs 26,5, protein 23

45) Thyme Zucchini Fries

Preparation Time: 10 minutes   **Cooking Time: 12 minutes**   **Servings:4**

Ingredients:

- 1 zucchini, thinly sliced
- A pinch of sea salt
- Black pepper to taste
- 1 teaspoon thyme, dried

- 1 egg
- 1 teaspoon garlic powder
- 1 cup almond flour

Directions:

⇒ In a bowl, whisk the egg with a pinch of salt.

⇒ Put the flour in another bowl and mix it with thyme, black pepper, and garlic powder.

⇒ Dredge zucchini slices in the egg mix and then in flour.

⇒ Arrange chips on a lined baking sheet, place in the oven at 450 degrees F and bake for 6 minutes on each side,

⇒ Serve the zucchini chips as a snack.

Nutrition: calories 106, fat 8,2, fiber 2,1, carbs 5,2, protein 5,1

46) Cheese Bites

Preparation Time: 5 minutes   **Cooking Time: 10 minutes**   **Servings: 24 pieces**

Ingredients:

- 1/3 cup tomatoes, chopped
- ½ cup bell peppers, mixed and chopped
- ½ cup tomato sauce

- 4 ounces almond cheese, cubed
- 2 tablespoons basil, chopped
- Black pepper to taste

Directions:

⇒ Divide tomato and bell pepper pieces into a muffin tray.

⇒ Also divide the tomato sauce, basil and almond cheese cubes, sprinkle black pepper at the end, place cups in the oven at 400 degrees F and bake for 10 minutes.

⇒ Arrange the meal on a platter and serve.

Nutrition: calories 59, fat 4,5, fiber 0,1, carbs 2, protein 2,5

47) Turkey Balls

Preparation Time: 10 minutes   **Cooking Time: 40 minutes**   **Servings:20**

Ingredients:

- 1 pound turkey meat, ground
- 1 tablespoon coconut oil, melted
- 1 yellow onion, chopped
- 1 egg
- 1 cup coconut flour

- 1 teaspoon Italian seasoning
- A pinch of sea salt
- Black pepper to taste
- 2 tablespoons parsley, chopped

Directions:

⇒ In a bowl, mix turkey meat with half of the flour, a pinch of salt, black pepper, Italian seasoning, parsley, onion, egg and hot sauce and stir well.

⇒ Put the rest of the flour in another bowl.

⇒ Shape 20 turkey meatballs and dip each one in flour.

⇒ Heat up a pan with the oil over medium-high heat, add meatballs, cook them for 4 minutes on each side, transfer to paper towels to remove any excess grease, place all of them on a platter and serve.

Nutrition: calories 71, fat 2,6, fiber 2,2, carbs 4,1, protein 7,7

48) Coconut Chicken Bites

Preparation Time: 10 minutes   **Cooking Time: 20 minutes**   **Servings:4**

Ingredients:

- 1 pound chicken tenders
- 1 egg, whisked
- A pinch of sea salt

- 1/3 cup coconut, unsweetened and shredded
- ¼ cup coconut flour

Directions:

⇒ In a bowl, mix coconut with coconut flour and a pinch of sea salt and stir.

⇒ Put whisked egg in another bowl.

⇒ Dip chicken pieces in egg, then in coconut mixture, arrange them all on a lined baking sheet and bake at 350 degrees F for 25 minutes.

⇒ Serve as a snack.

Nutrition: calories 330, fat 13,6, fiber 8,1, carbs 13,6, protein 36,9

49) Dehydrated Beef Bites

Preparation Time: 6 hours   **Cooking Time: 6 hours**   **Servings:6**

Ingredients:

- ½ cup coconut aminos
- 2 and ½ pounds beef, thinly sliced
- 2 tablespoons gluten free liquid smoke

- ¼ cup coconut sugar
- ¼ cup apple cider vinegar
- A pinch of sea salt

Directions:

⇒ In a bowl, mix vinegar with coconut sugar, aminos, liquid smoke, ginger and a pinch of salt and stir well.

⇒ Add meat slices, toss to coat well, cover and keep in the fridge for 6 hours.

⇒ Transfer meat slices to your preheated dehydrator at 165 degrees F and dehydrate them for 6 hours.

⇒ Transfer beef jerky to a bowl and serve as a snack.

Nutrition: calories 273, fat 8,3, fiber 0, carbs 12,9, protein 33,3

50) Chicken Platter

Preparation Time: 3 hours   **Cooking Time: 15 minutes**   **Servings:4**

Ingredients:

- 2 tablespoons parsley, chopped
- 4 chicken breasts, cubed

- ¾ cup garlic powder
- Black pepper to taste

Directions:

⇒ In a bowl, mix chicken with garlic powder, black pepper, and parsley, stir well, cover and keep in the fridge for 3 hours.

⇒ Arrange chicken pieces on skewers, place them all on preheated grill and cook for 15 minutes, flipping once.

⇒ Arrange skewers on a platter and serve as an appetizer.

Nutrition: calories 485, fat 22,9, fiber 2,6, carbs 18,6, protein 53,1

51) Baked Kale Bowls

Preparation Time: 10 minutes   **Cooking Time: 20 minutes**   **Servings:6**

Ingredients:

- 1 tablespoon avocado oil
- 1 bunch kale, leaves separated

- A pinch of sea salt
- Black pepper to taste

Directions:

⇒ Pat dry kale leaves, arrange them on a lined baking sheet, drizzle the oil, sprinkle a pinch of sea salt and black pepper to taste, place in the oven at 275 degrees F and bake for 20 minutes.

⇒ Serve the chips cold.

Nutrition: calories 9, fat 0,3, fiber 0,3, carbs 1,3, protein 0,4

52) Herbed Snack

Preparation Time: 10 minutes   **Cooking Time: 14 minutes**   **Servings:40**

Ingredients:

- ¼ cup coconut flour
- 1 cup almond flour
- ½ cup sesame seeds, toasted and ground
- 2 tablespoons tapioca flour
- A pinch of sea salt

- Black pepper to taste
- 1 teaspoon onion powder
- 1 teaspoon rosemary, chopped
- ½ teaspoon thyme, chopped
- 2 eggs
- 3 tablespoons olive oil

Directions:

⇒ In a bowl, mix sesame seeds with coconut flour, almond flour, tapioca flour, salt, pepper, rosemary, thyme and onion powder and stir well.

⇒ In another bowl, whisk eggs with the oil and stir well.

⇒ Add this to flour mix and knead until you obtain a dough.

⇒ Shape a disk out of this dough, flatten well and cut 40 crackers out of it.

⇒ Arrange them all on a lined baking sheet, place in the oven at 375 degrees F and bake for 14 minutes.

⇒ Leave your crackers to cool down and serve them as a snack.

Nutrition: calories 37, fat 2,9, fiber 1,1, carbs 2,2, protein 1,1

53) Pumpkin Crakers

Preparation Time: 10 minutes   **Cooking Time: 3 hours**   **Servings:40**

Ingredients:

- ½ cup chia seeds
- 1 cup flaxseed, ground
- ½ cup pumpkin seeds
- 1/3 cup sesame seeds
- A pinch of sea salt

- 1 and ¼ cups water
- ½ teaspoon garlic powder
- 1 teaspoon thyme, dried
- 1 teaspoon basil, dried

Directions:

⇒ Put pumpkin seeds in your food processor, pulse well and transfer them to a bowl.

⇒ Add flaxseed, sesame seeds, chia, salt, water, garlic powder, thyme and basil and stir well until they combine.

⇒ Spread this on a lined baking sheet, press well, cuts into 40 pieces, place in the oven at 200 degrees F and bake for 3 hours.

⇒ Leave your crackers to cool down before serving them as a snack.

Nutrition: calories 35, fat 2,5, fiber 1,2, carbs 1,7, protein 1,3

54) Cashew Crackers

Preparation Time: 30 minutes   **Cooking Time: 0 minutes**   **Servings:10**

Ingredients:

- 1 teaspoon vanilla extract
- 1 cup coconut flakes, unsweetened
- 2 cups cashews
- 1 and ¼ cups figs, dried

- A pinch of sea salt
- 1/3 cup cocoa butter
- ¾ cup cocoa powder
- 1 tablespoon cocoa powder

Directions:

⇒ In your food processor, mix figs with vanilla, cashews, a pinch of salt, cocoa powder and coconut and blend them well.

⇒ Transfer this into a baking dish and press well.

⇒ Put cocoa powder and cocoa butter in a heatproof bowl, place in your microwave for 3 minutes until it melts.

⇒ Pour this over coconut mix, spread well, place in your freezer for 20 minutes, cut into crackers and serve as a snack.

Nutrition: calories 1504, fat 28,1, fiber 52,2, carbs 331,5, protein 22,1

Chapter 6 -   Meat Recipes

55) Salsa Pork Mix

Preparation Time: 12 hours and 10 minutes | **Cooking Time: 8 hours and 20 minutes** | **Servings:4**

Ingredients:

- ½ cup paleo salsa
- ½ cup beef stock
- ½ cup enchilada sauce
- 3 pounds organic pork shoulder
- 2 green chilies, chopped
- 1 tablespoon garlic powder
- 1 tablespoon chili powder
- 1 teaspoon onion powder
- 1 teaspoon cumin, ground
- 1 teaspoon sweet paprika
- Black pepper to taste

Directions:

⇒ In a bowl, mix chili powder with onion and garlic one.

⇒ Add cumin, paprika and pepper to taste and stir everything.

⇒ Add pork, rub well and keep in the fridge for 12 hours.

⇒ Transfer pork to a slow cooker, add enchilada sauce, stock, salsa and green chilies, stir, cover and cook on Low for 8 hours.

⇒ Transfer pork to a plate, leave aside to cool down and shred.

⇒ Strain sauce from slow cooker into a pan, bring to a boil over medium heat and simmer for 8 minutes stirring all the time.

⇒ Add shredded pork to the sauce, stir, reduce heat to medium and cook for 20 more minutes.

⇒ Divide between plates and serve hot.

Nutrition: calories 1013, fat 73, carbs 4,3, fiber 1,6, protein 80,4

56) Smoked Pork Ribs

Preparation Time: 15 minutes | **Cooking Time: 2 hours and 47 minutes** | **Servings:4**

Ingredients:

- 1 tablespoon smoked paprika
- ½ tablespoon onion powder
- ½ tablespoon garlic powder
- ½ teaspoon cayenne pepper
- 4 pounds baby ribs
- 1 cup paleo BBQ sauce
- 4 teaspoons Sriracha
- ¼ cup cilantro, chopped
- ¼ cup chives, chopped
- ¼ cup parsley, chopped
- Black pepper to taste

Directions:

⇒ In a bowl, mix paprika with onion powder, garlic powder, pepper and cayenne and stir well.

⇒ Add ribs, toss to coat and arrange them on a lined baking sheet.

⇒ Place in the oven at 325 degrees F and bake them for 2 hours and 30 minutes.

⇒ In a bowl, mix BBQ sauce with Sriracha and stir well.

⇒ Take ribs out of the oven, mix them with BBQ sauce, place them on preheated grill over medium-high heat and cook for 7 minutes on each side.

⇒ Divide ribs between plates, sprinkle chives, cilantro, and parsley on top and serve.

Nutrition: calories 1483, fat 122,3, fiber 1,1, carbs 9,5, protein 81,8

57) Sage Pork

Preparation Time: 10 minutes   **Cooking Time: 30 minutes**   **Servings:4**

Ingredients:

- 8 sage springs
- 4 pork chops, bone-in
- 4 tablespoons ghee
- 4 garlic cloves, crushed

- 1 tablespoon coconut oil
- A pinch of sea salt
- Black pepper to taste

Directions:

⇒ Season pork chops with a pinch of sea salt and pepper to taste.

⇒ Heat up a pan with the oil over medium high heat, add pork chops and cook for 10 minutes turning them often.

⇒ Take pork chops off heat, add ghee, sage, and garlic and toss to coat.

⇒ Return to heat, cook for 4 minutes often stirring, divide between plates and serve.

Nutrition: calories 402, fat 36, fiber 0,1, carbs 1, protein 18,2

58) Balsamic Pork Mix

Preparation Time: 10 minutes   **Cooking Time: 45 minutes**   **Servings:4**

Ingredients:

- 1 yellow onion, chopped
- 1 organic pork tenderloin
- 2 pears, chopped
- 2 garlic cloves, minced
- 1 tablespoon chives, chopped
- ¼ cup walnuts, chopped

- 3 tablespoons balsamic vinegar
- Black pepper to taste
- ½ cup chicken stock
- 1 tablespoon coconut oil
- 1 tablespoon lemon juice

Directions:

⇒ In a bowl, mix walnuts with pear, chives, pepper and lemon juice and stir well.

⇒ Heat up a pan with the oil over medium-high heat, add tenderloin and brown for 3 minutes on each side.

⇒ Reduce heat, add onion and garlic, stir and cook for 2 minutes.

⇒ Add balsamic vinegar, stock, pear mix, stir, place in the oven at 400 degrees F and bake for 20 minutes.

⇒ Take pork out of the oven, leave aside for 4 minutes, slice, divide between plates and serve with pear salsa on top.

Nutrition: calories 271, fat 11,2, fiber 4,4, carbs 20,1, protein 24,6

59) Pork with Carrots and Sauce

Preparation Time: 10 minutes   **Cooking Time: 45 minutes**   **Servings:4**

Ingredients:

- 15 oz turkey mince
- A handful arugula
- Black pepper to taste
- 1 grass fed pork tenderloin
- 1 tablespoon coconut oil

  For the puree:
- 1 sweet potato, chopped
- 3 carrots, chopped
- A pinch of sea salt

- Black pepper to taste
- 1 tablespoon curry paste

  For the sauce:
- 2 tablespoons balsamic vinegar
- 1 teaspoon mustard
- 2 shallots, chopped
- Black pepper to taste
- 4 tablespoons extra virgin olive oil

Directions:

⇒ Slice pork tenderloin in half horizontally but not all the way and open it up.

⇒ Use a meat tenderizer to even it up.

⇒ Place turkey mince in the middle, roll pork around it, tie with twine, season pepper to taste and leave to one side.

⇒ Heat up an oven proof pan with the coconut oil over medium-high heat, add pork roll, cook for 3 minutes on each side, place in the oven at 350 degrees F and bake for 25 minutes.

⇒ Meanwhile, put potatoes and carrots in a large saucepan, add water to cover, bring to a boil over medium-high heat, cook for 20 minutes, drain and transfer to a food processor.

⇒ Pulse a few times until you obtain a puree, add a pinch of sea salt and pepper to taste, blend again, transfer to a bowl and leave aside.

⇒ Take pork roll out of the oven, slice and divide between plates.

⇒ Heat up a pan with the olive oil over medium-high heat, add shallots, stir and cook for 10 minutes.

⇒ Add balsamic vinegar, mustard, pepper, stir well and take off heat. Divide carrots puree next to pork slices, drizzle vinegar sauce on to and serve with arugula on the side.

Nutrition: calories 495, fat 29,5, carbs 2,2, fiber 17,5, protein 21,8

60) Garlic Pork and Strawberries

Preparation Time: 10 minutes   **Cooking Time: 35 minutes**   **Servings:4**

Ingredients:

- 4 pounds pork tenderloin
- 1 cup strawberries, sliced
- 10 thin turkey fillet strips
- A pinch of sea salt

- Black pepper to taste
- 4 garlic cloves, minced
- ½ cup balsamic vinegar
- 2 tablespoons extra virgin olive oil

Directions:

⇒ Wrap turkey strips around tenderloin, secure with toothpicks and season with salt and pepper.

⇒ Heat up your grill over indirect medium high heat, put tenderloin on it and cook for 30 minutes.

⇒ Heat up a pan with the oil over medium high heat, add garlic, stir and cook for 2 minutes.

⇒ Add vinegar and half of the strawberries, stir and bring to a boil.

⇒ Reduce heat to medium and simmer for 10 minutes.

⇒ Add black pepper to taste and the rest of the strawberries and stir.

⇒ Baste pork with some of the sauce and continue cooking over indirect heat until turkey is brown enough.

⇒ Transfer pork to a cutting board, leave aside for a few minutes to cool down, slice and divide between plates.

⇒ Serve with the strawberry sauce right away.

Nutrition: calories 981, fat 24,3, carbs 4, fiber 0,8, protein 174,1

61) Turkey with Peppers and Tomatoes

Preparation Time: 15 minutes   **Cooking Time: 45 minutes**   **Servings:6**

Ingredients:

- 20 ounces ground turkey
- 2 green bell peppers, chopped
- 3 sweet potatoes, chopped
- 1-pint grape tomatoes, chopped
- A pinch of sea salt

- Black pepper to taste
- 2 garlic cloves, minced
- 1 red onion, chopped
- A few thyme springs

Directions:

⇒ In a baking dish, mix potatoes with tomatoes, onion, bell pepper, garlic, a pinch of sea salt and pepper and stir gently.

⇒ Heat up a pan over high heat, add turkey mince, brown it for 15 minutes side and transfer on top of veggies in the baking dish.

⇒ Add thyme, introduce in the oven at 400 degrees F and bake for 45 minutes.

⇒ Divide between plates and serve hot.

Nutrition: calories 306, fat 10,8, carbs 28,4, fiber 4,8, protein 28,2

62) Steak and Veggies

Preparation Time: 10 minutes   **Cooking Time: 20 minutes**   **Servings:4**

Ingredients:

- 3 sweet potatoes, cubed
- 1 yellow onion, chopped
- 12 mini bell peppers, chopped
- 4 medium round steaks
- ½ cup sun dried tomatoes, chopped
- 1 tablespoon sweet paprika
- 2 tablespoons balsamic vinegar
- Juice of 1 lemon

- 1 tablespoons oregano, dried
- ¼ cup olive oil+ a drizzle
- 1 lemon, sliced
- ¼ cup kalamata olives, pitted and chopped
- 4 dill springs
- 2 garlic cloves, minced
- A pinch of sea salt and black pepper

Directions:

⇒ Heat up a pan with a drizzle of oil over medium-high heat, add steaks, season them with salt and some black pepper, brown them for 2 minutes on each side and transfer to a baking dish.

⇒ Heat up the pan again over medium-high heat, add sweet potatoes, cook them for 4 minutes and add them to the baking dish.

⇒ Also add bell peppers, tomatoes, onion, olives and lemon slices.

⇒ Meanwhile, in a bowl, mix lemon juice with rest of the olive oil, vinegar, garlic, paprika and oregano and whisk well.

⇒ Pour this over steak and veggies, add dill springs on top, toss to coat, place in the oven at 425 degrees F and bake for 12 minutes.

⇒ Divide steak and veggies between plates and serve.

Nutrition: calories 869, fat 30,8, fiber 10,9, carbs 56,5, protein 89,1

63) Steaks and Pico de Gallo

Preparation Time: 10 minutes   **Cooking Time: 15 minutes**   **Servings:4**

Ingredients:

- 2 tablespoons chili powder
- 4 medium sirloin steaks
- 1 teaspoon cumin, ground
- ½ tablespoon sweet paprika
- 1 teaspoon onion powder
- 1 teaspoon garlic powder
- A pinch of sea salt and black pepper

For the Pico de gallo:

- 1 small red onion, chopped

- 2 tomatoes, chopped
- 2 garlic cloves, minced
- 2 tablespoons lime juice
- 1 small green bell pepper, chopped
- 1 jalapeno, chopped
- ¼ cup cilantro, chopped
- ¼ teaspoon cumin, ground
- Black pepper to taste

Directions:

⇒ In a bowl, mix chili powder with a pinch of salt, black pepper, onion powder, garlic powder, paprika and 1 teaspoon cumin and stir well.

⇒ Season steaks with this mix, rub well and place them on preheated grill over medium high heat.

⇒ Cook steaks for 5 minutes on each side and divide them between plates.

⇒ In a bowl, mix red onion with tomatoes, garlic, lime juice, bell pepper, jalapeno, cilantro, black pepper to taste and ¼ teaspoon cumin and stir well.

⇒ Top steaks with this mix and serve.

Nutrition: calories 285, fat 9, fiber 3,1 carbs 10,2, protein 40,5

64) Coffee Steaks

Preparation Time: 10 minutes   **Cooking Time: 10 minutes**   **Servings:4**

Ingredients:

- 1 and ½ tablespoons coffee, ground
- 4 rib eye steaks
- ½ tablespoon sweet paprika
- 2 tablespoons chili powder
- 2 teaspoons garlic powder

- 2 teaspoons onion powder
- ¼ teaspoon ginger, ground
- ¼ teaspoon, coriander, ground
- A pinch of cayenne pepper
- Black pepper to the taste

Directions:

⇒ In a bowl, mix coffee with paprika, chili powder, garlic powder, onion powder, ginger, coriander, cayenne and black pepper and stir well.

⇒ Rub steaks with the coffee mix, place them on your preheated grill over medium high heat, cook them for 5 minutes on each side and divide between plates.

⇒ Leave steaks to cool down for 5 minutes before serving them with a side salad!

Nutrition: calories 621, fat 50, fiber 0, carbs 0, protein 40

65) Beef Casserolle

Preparation Time: 10 minutes   **Cooking Time: 6 hours**   **Servings:6**

Ingredients:

- 1 red bell pepper, chopped
- 1 eggplant, sliced lengthwise
- 2 zucchinis, sliced lengthwise
- 1 pound beef, ground
- 2 cups tomatoes, chopped
- 2 teaspoons oregano, dried
- 4 cups tomato sauce
- ¼ cup basil, chopped

- 2 garlic cloves, minced
- 1 yellow onion, chopped
- 2 tablespoons tomato paste
- 1 tablespoon parsley, chopped
- 2 tablespoons olive oil
- A pinch of sea salt
- Black pepper to taste

Directions:

⇒ Heat up a pan with the oil over medium-high heat, add onion and garlic, stir and cook for 2 minutes.

⇒ Add beef, stir and brown for 5 minutes more.

⇒ Add bell pepper, tomatoes, oregano, basil, tomato paste and parsley, stir and cook for 4 minutes more.

⇒ Add tomato sauce, black pepper to taste and a pinch of salt and stir well again.

⇒ Arrange layers of eggplant and zucchini slices with the sauce you've made in your slow cooker.

⇒ Cover and cook on Low for 4 hours and 45 minutes.

⇒ Divide your lasagna between plates and serve.

Nutrition: calories 281, fat 10,2, fiber 7,7, carbs 22,7, protein 28

Chapter 7 -   Seafood & Fish Recipes

66) Sesame Tuna

Preparation Time: 15 minutes   **Cooking Time: 10 minutes**   **Servings:4**

Ingredients:

- 1 teaspoon fennel seeds
- 1 teaspoon mustard seeds
- 4 medium tuna steaks
- ¼ teaspoon black peppercorns

- A pinch of sea salt
- Black pepper to taste
- 4 tablespoons sesame seeds, toasted
- 3 tablespoons coconut oil, melted

Directions:

⇒ In your grinder, mix peppercorns with fennel, mustard seeds, sesame seeds, a pinch of sea salt, pepper to taste and grind well.

⇒ Spread this mix on a plate, add tuna steaks and toss to coat.

⇒ Heat up a pan with the oil over medium-high heat, add tuna steaks and cook for 3 minutes on each side.

⇒ Divide between plates and serve with a side salad.

Nutrition: calories 458, fat 25,7, carbs 2,7, fiber 1,4, protein 52,8

67) Lime Tartar

Preparation Time: 15 minutes   **Cooking Time: 0 minutes**   **Servings:4**

Ingredients:

- 7 ounces smoked salmon, minced
- 14 ounces salmon fillet, cut into very small cubes
- 3 tablespoons red onion, minced
- 2 tablespoons pickled cucumber, minced
- Zest and juice from 1 lemon
- 1 garlic clove, finely minced
- 2 tablespoons basil, minced

- 2 teaspoons oregano, dried
- Black pepper to taste
- 2 tablespoons mint leaves, minced
- 2 tablespoons Dijon mustard
- 5 tablespoons extra virgin olive oil
- Lime wedges for serving

Directions:

⇒ In a bowl, combine all the ingredients, stir well and keep in the fridge for 15 minutes

⇒ Divide the tartar between plates and serve with lime wedges on the side.

Nutrition: calories 361, fat 26,3, carbs 5,1, fiber 1,5, protein 29,2

68) Salmon and Onion Mix

Preparation Time: 10 minutes   **Cooking Time: 15 minutes**   **Servings:4**

Ingredients:

- 2 red onions, cut into wedges
- 3 peaches, cut into wedges
- 4 salmon steaks
- 1 teaspoon thyme, chopped
- 1 tablespoon ginger, grated

- A pinch of sea salt
- Black pepper to taste
- 1 tablespoon balsamic vinegar
- 3 tablespoons extra virgin olive oil

Directions:

⇒ In a bowl, mix the ginger, vinegar, thyme, a pinch of sea salt, pepper and olive oil and whisk very well.

⇒ In another bowl, mix peaches with onion, salt and pepper and toss to coat.

⇒ Heat up your kitchen grill over medium-high heat, add salmon steaks, season with salt and pepper, grill for 6 minutes on each side and divide between plates.

⇒ Add peaches and onions to grill, cook for 4 minutes on each side and transfer next to salmon on plates.

⇒ Drizzle the vinaigrette you've made all over the salmon and peaches mix and serve.

Nutrition: calories 398, fat 22, carbs 16,8, fiber 3,2, protein 36,3

69) Shrimp and Radish Cakes

Preparation Time: 15 minutes　　　　**Cooking Time: 15 minutes**　　　　**Servings:4**

Ingredients:

- 2 tablespoons cilantro, chopped
- 1 and ½ pounds shrimp, peeled and deveined
- 2 tablespoons chives, chopped
- Black pepper to taste
- 1 garlic clove, minced
- ¼ cup radishes, minced
- 1 teaspoon lemon zest, grated
- ¼ cup celery, minced
- 1 egg, whisked
- 1 tablespoon lemon juice
- ¼ cup almond meal

For the salsa:

- 1 avocado, pitted, peeled and chopped
- 1 cup pineapple, chopped
- 2 tablespoons red onion, chopped
- ¼ cup bell peppers, chopped
- 1 tablespoon lime juice
- 1 tablespoon cilantro, finely chopped
- A pinch of sea salt
- Black pepper to taste

Directions:

⇒ In a bowl, mix the pineapple with avocado, bell peppers, 2 tablespoons red onion, 1 tablespoon lime juice, pepper to taste and 1 tablespoon cilantro, stir well and keep in the fridge for now.

⇒ In your food processor, mix shrimp with 2 tablespoons cilantro, chives, and garlic and blend well.

⇒ Transfer to a bowl and mix with radishes, celery, lemon zest, lemon juice, egg, almond meal, a pinch of sea salt and pepper to taste and stir well.

⇒ Shape 4 burgers, place them on preheated grill over medium-high heat and cook for 5 minutes on each side.

⇒ Divide shrimp burgers between plates and serve with the salsa you've made earlier on the side.

Nutrition:　　　　calories 406, fat 17,2, carbs 16,1, fiber 5,3, protein 46,8

70) Basil Scallops Mix

Preparation Time: 15 minutes　　　　**Cooking Time: 0 minutes**　　　　**Servings:2**

Ingredients:

- 6 scallops, diced
- A pinch of sea salt
- Black pepper to taste
- 3 strawberries, chopped
- 1 tablespoon extra-virgin olive oil
- 1 tablespoon green onions, minced
- Juice from ½ lemon
- ½ tablespoon basil leaves, finely chopped

Directions:

⇒ In a bowl, mix all the ingredients, toss and keep in the fridge for 15 minutes.

⇒ Keep the tartar in the fridge until ready to serve.

Nutrition:　　　　calories 149, fat 7,8, carbs 4,8, fiber 0,5, protein 15,3

71) Creole Shrimp Mix

Preparation Time: 10 minutes   **Cooking Time: 10 minutes**   Servings:4

Ingredients:

- ½ pound turkey meat, already cooked and sliced
- ½ pound shrimp, peeled and deveined
- 2 tablespoons extra virgin olive oil
- 2 zucchinis, cubed
- A pinch of sea salt
- Black pepper to taste

For the Creole seasoning:

- ½ tablespoon garlic powder
- 2 tablespoons paprika
- ½ tablespoon onion powder
- ¼ tablespoon oregano, dried
- ½ tablespoon chili powder
- ¼ tablespoon thyme, dried

Directions:

⇒ In a bowl, mix paprika with garlic powder, onion one, chili powder, oregano, and thyme and stir well.

⇒ In another bowl, mix shrimp with turkey meat, zucchini, and oil and toss to coat.

⇒ Pour paprika mix over shrimp mix and stir well.

⇒ Arrange turkey, shrimp, and zucchini on skewers alternating pieces, season with a pinch of sea salt and black pepper, place them on preheated grill over medium-high heat and cook for 8 minutes, flipping skewers from time to time.

⇒ Divide the skewers between plates and serve.

Nutrition: calories 260, fat 11,7, fiber 3, carbs 8,3, protein 31,7

72) Orange Salmon Bites

Preparation Time: 10 minutes   **Cooking Time: 15 minutes**   Servings:4

Ingredients:

- 1 pound wild salmon, skinless, boneless and cubed
- 2 Meyer lemons, sliced
- ¼ cup balsamic vinegar

- ¼ cup orange juice
- A pinch of pink salt
- Black pepper to taste

Directions:

⇒ Heat up a small saucepan with the vinegar over medium heat, add the orange juice, stir, bring to a simmer for 1 minute and take off the heat.

⇒ Skewer salmon cubes and lemon slices, season with salt and black pepper, brush them with half of the vinegar mix, place on preheated grill over medium heat, cook for 4 minutes on each side.

⇒ Brush skewers with the rest of the vinegar mix, grill for 1 minute more, divide between plates and serve.

Nutrition: calories 290, fat 12,6, fiber 3, carbs 11,8, protein 40,3

73) Sushi Tuna Mix

Preparation Time: 10 minutes   **Cooking Time: 5 minutes**   **Servings:4**

Ingredients:

- 1 small red onion, chopped
- ½ cup cilantro, chopped
- 1/3 cup olive oil+ 2 tablespoons
- 1 jalapeno pepper, chopped
- 2 tablespoons basil, chopped
- 3 tablespoons vinegar
- 3 garlic cloves, minced

- 1 teaspoon red pepper flakes
- 1 teaspoon thyme, chopped
- A pinch of sea salt
- Black pepper to taste
- 1 pound sushi grade tuna
- 2 avocados, pitted, peeled and chopped
- 6 ounces arugula

Directions:

⇒ In a bowl, mix 1/3 cup oil with onion, jalapeno, cilantro, basil, vinegar, garlic, parsley, pepper flakes, thyme, a pinch of salt and black pepper and whisk well.

⇒ Heat up a pan with the rest of the oil over medium-high heat, add tuna, season salt and black pepper, cook for 2 minutes on each side, transfer to a cutting board, leave aside to cool down and slice.

⇒ In a bowl, mix arugula with half of the chimichurri sauce you've made earlier, toss to coat well and divide between plates.

⇒ Also divide tuna slices, and avocado pieces and drizzle the rest of the sauce on top.

Nutrition: calories 938, fat 62,8, fiber 10, carbs 51,9, protein 43,8

74) Chili Salmon

Preparation Time: 10 minutes   **Cooking Time: 15 minutes**   **Servings:12**

Ingredients:

- 1 and ¼ cups coconut, shredded
- 1 pound salmon meat, cubed
- 1/3 cup coconut flour
- A pinch of sea salt
- Black pepper to taste
- 1 egg

- 2 tablespoons coconut oil
- ¼ cup water
- 4 red chilies, chopped
- 3 garlic cloves, minced
- ¼ cup balsamic vinegar
- ½ cup honey

Directions:

⇒ In another bowl, whisk the egg with black pepper.

⇒ Put coconut in a third bowl.

⇒ Dip salmon cubes in flour, egg and coconut and place them all on a working surface.

⇒ Heat up a pan with the oil over medium-high heat, add salmon cubes, fry them for 3 minutes on each side, transfer them to paper towels, drain grease and divide them between plates.

⇒ Heat up a pan with the water over medium-high heat.

⇒ Add chilies, cloves, vinegar, honey and agar agar, stir well, bring to a gentle boil and simmer until all ingredients combine.

⇒ Drizzle this over salmon cubes and serve.

Nutrition: calories 180, fat 8,5, fiber 0,9, carbs 19,7, protein 7,7

75) Clams and Apple Mix

Preparation Time: 10 minutes   **Cooking Time: 12 minutes**   **Servings:2**

Ingredients:

- 3 tablespoons ghee, melted
- 2 pound little clams, scrubbed
- 1 shallot, minced
- 2 garlic cloves, minced

- 1 cup cider
- 1 apple, cored and chopped
- Juice of ½ lemon

Directions:

⇒ Heat up a pan with the ghee over medium-high heat, add the shallot and garlic, stir and cook for 3 minutes.

⇒ Add cider, stir well and cook for 1 minute.

⇒ Add clams and thyme, cover and simmer for 5 minutes.

⇒ Add apple and lemon juice, stir, divide everything into bowls and serve.

Nutrition: calories 610, fat 23,6, fiber 2,9, carbs 43,7, protein 55,1

76) Fennel Salmon Mix

Preparation Time: 10 minutes   **Cooking Time: 30 minutes**   **Servings:6**

Ingredients:

- 2 tablespoons ghee, melted
- A pinch of sea salt
- Black pepper to taste
- 3 cups chicken stock

- ½ teaspoon fennel seeds
- 1 teaspoon mustard seeds
- 2 apples, cored, peeled and cubed
- 4 salmon fillets, skin on and bone in

Directions:

⇒ Put the stock in a pot, heat up over medium heat, add mustard seeds, a pinch of salt, black pepper and fennel seeds, stir and boil for 25 minutes.

⇒ Strain this into a bowl, add half of the ghee, stir well and leave aside for now.

⇒ Heat up a pan with the rest of the ghee over medium heat, add apple pieces, stir and cook for 6 minutes.

⇒ Brush salmon pieces with some of the stock mix, season with a pinch of salt and black pepper, place on a lined baking sheet, also add apple pieces, introduce everything in the oven at 350 degrees F and bake for 25 minutes.

⇒ Divide salmon between plates and serve with the rest of the stock drizzled on top.

Nutrition: calories 241, fat 12,2, fiber 2, carbs 10,9, protein 23,7

77) Shrimp and Parsley Mix

Preparation Time: 10 minutes   **Cooking Time: 5 minutes**   **Servings:4**

Ingredients:

- 1 pound big shrimp, peeled and deveined
- 2 teaspoons olive oil
- 1 cup cilantro, chopped
- 1 cup parsley, chopped
- Juice from 2 limes

- ½ cup olive oil
- ¼ cup yellow onion, chopped
- A pinch of sea salt
- ½ teaspoon smoked paprika
- 2 garlic cloves, minced

Directions:

⇒ Heat up a pan with 2 teaspoons olive oil over medium heat, add shrimp, cook them for 5 minutes and reduce heat to low.

⇒ In a food processor, mix ½ cup oil with onion, sea salt, paprika, garlic, lime juice, parsley and cilantro and pulse well.

⇒ Divide shrimp on plates, top with the chimichurri and serve.

Nutrition: calories 374, fat 26,9, fiber 1, carbs 4,3, protein 30,5

78) Scallops Salad

Preparation Time: 10 minutes   **Cooking Time: 13 minutes**   **Servings:4**

Ingredients:

- 1 shallot, minced
- 3 garlic cloves, minced
- 1 and ½ cups chicken stock
- ¼ cup walnuts, toasted and chopped
- 1 and ½ cups grapes, halved
- 2 cups spinach
- 1 tablespoon avocado oil
- 1 pound scallops
- A pinch of sea salt
- Black pepper to taste

Directions:

⇒ Heat up a pan with the oil over medium heat, add the shallot and the garlic, stir and cook for 2 minutes.

⇒ Add the walnuts, grapes, salt and pepper, stir and cook for 3 more minutes.

⇒ Add the scallops and cook them for 2 minutes on each side.

⇒ Add the spinach, toss, cook everything for 3 more minutes, divide everything into bowls and serve.

Nutrition: calories 205, fat 7,4, fiber 1,5, carbs 17,5, protein 24,9

79) Crab and Sauce

Preparation Time: 10 minutes   **Cooking Time: 7 minutes**   **Servings:8**

Ingredients:

- 1 cup crab meat
- 2 tablespoons parsley, chopped
- 2 tablespoons old bay seasoning
- 2 teaspoons Dijon mustard
- 1 egg, whisked
- 1 tablespoons lemon juice
- 2 tablespoons coconut oil
- 1 and ½ tablespoons coconut flour

For the sauce:

- 1 tablespoon olive oil
- ¼ cup roasted red peppers
- 1 tablespoon lemon juice
- ¼ cup avocado, peeled and chopped

Directions:

⇒ In a bowl, mix crabmeat with old bay seasoning, parsley, mustard, egg, 1 tablespoon lemon juice and coconut flour and stir everything very well.

⇒ Shape 8 patties from this mix and place them on a plate.

⇒ Heat up a pan with 2 tablespoons coconut oil over medium-high heat, add crab patties, cook for 3 minutes on each side and divide between plates.

⇒ In a food processor, mix olive oil with red peppers, avocado and 1 tablespoon lemon juice and blend well.

⇒ Spread this on the crab patties and serve.

Nutrition: calories 69, fat 6,8, fiber 0,5, carbs 1,1, protein 1,4

Chapter 8 -   Salad Recipes

80) Broccoli and Beef Salad

Preparation Time: 10 minutes   **Cooking Time: 10 minutes**   **Servings:4**

Ingredients:

- 1 pound organic beef steak, cut into strips
- 3 cups broccoli, florets separated
- 8 cups baby salad greens
- 1 red onion, sliced
- 1 red bell pepper, sliced

For the vinaigrette:

- 1 tablespoon ginger, minced

- A pinch of sea salt
- Black pepper to taste
- ½ cup extra virgin olive oil
- 2 tablespoons lime juice
- 1 tablespoon balsamic vinegar
- 2 tablespoons shallots, finely chopped

Directions:

⇒ In a bowl, mix ginger with oil, lime juice, vinegar, shallots, a pinch of sea salt and pepper to taste and stir well.

⇒ Heat up a pan over medium-high heat, add 2 tablespoons of vinaigrette, warm up, add broccoli and cook for 3 minutes.

⇒ Add beef, stir and cook for 4 more minutes and take off heat.

⇒ In a salad bowl, mix salad greens with onion, bell pepper, broccoli, and beef.

⇒ Add some black pepper, drizzle the rest of the vinaigrette, toss to coat and serve.

Nutrition: calories 513, fat 32,7, carbs 17,6, fiber 5, protein 39,2

81) Dijon Spinach Salad

Preparation Time: 10 minutes   **Cooking Time: 20 minutes**   **Servings:4**

Ingredients:

- 2 red onions, cut into medium wedges
- 1 butternut squash, cut into medium wedges
- 6 cups spinach
- 4 parsnips, cut into medium wedges
- Black pepper to taste
- 2 tablespoons balsamic vinegar

- 1/3 cup nuts, roasted
- 1 teaspoon Dijon mustard
- ½ tablespoons oregano, dried
- 1 garlic clove, minced
- 6 tablespoons extra virgin olive oil

Directions:

⇒ Put the squash, onions, and parsnips in a baking dish.

⇒ Drizzle half of the oil, sprinkle oregano and pepper to the taste, toss to coat, place in the oven at 400 degrees F and bake for 10 minutes.

⇒ Take veggies out of the oven, turn them and bake for another 10 minutes.

⇒ In a bowl, mix vinegar with the rest of the oil, garlic, mustard and pepper to taste and stir very well.

⇒ Put spinach in a salad bowl, add roasted veggies, pour salad dressing, sprinkle nuts, toss to coat and serve warm.

Nutrition: calories 401, fat 27,7, carbs 38,4, fiber 10,7, protein 6

82) Chicken and Arugula Salad

Preparation Time: 10 minutes   **Cooking Time: 35 minutes**   **Servings:4**

Ingredients:

- 2 tablespoons ghee, melted
- 1 tablespoon balsamic vinegar
- 1 zucchini, cubed
- 2 small shallots, peeled, chopped
- 4 eggs
- 2 lettuce heads, leaves, torn
- 2 cups chicken meat, already cooked and shredded
- 4 cups arugula
- 1 small red onion, finely chopped
- 1/3 cup cranberries
- A pinch of sea salt

- Black pepper to taste
- A pinch of garlic powder
- 1/3 cup pecans, chopped
- 2 apples, chopped
- 2 tablespoons maple syrup
- 1 tablespoon apple cider vinegar
- 1 teaspoon shallot, minced
- 1 teaspoon mustard
- 1 teaspoon garlic, minced
- ¼ cup extra virgin olive oil

Directions:

⇒ Spread zucchini cubes on a lined baking sheet, sprinkle with a pinch of sea salt, pepper, garlic powder, drizzle balsamic vinegar and add ghee, toss to coat, place in the oven at 400 degrees F and bake for 25 minutes.

⇒ Meanwhile, put eggs in a saucepan, add water to cover, bring to a boil over medium-high heat, boil for 15 minutes, drain, place in a bowl filled with ice water, leave aside to cool down, peel them, chop and put in a salad bowl. Heat up a pan over medium-high heat, add shallots, brown for 7 minutes, take off heat, leave to cool down and add to the same bowl with the eggs.

⇒ Add lettuce leaves, arugula, chicken, onion, pecans, apple pieces, roasted squash cubes, and cranberries. In a small bowl, mix maple syrup with apple cider vinegar, mustard, garlic, shallot, olive oil and pepper and whisk very well.

⇒ Pour this over salad, toss to coat and serve.

Nutrition: calories 628, fat 42, carbs 36,9, fiber 7,3, protein 30,5

83) Cayenne Scallops and Avocado Salad

Preparation Time: 10 minutes   **Cooking Time: 7 minutes**   **Servings:4**

Ingredients:

- 1 pound bay scallops
- 2 teaspoons cayenne pepper
- Black pepper to taste
- 3 tablespoons lemon juice
- 1 tablespoon homemade mayonnaise
- 1 teaspoon mustard
- A pinch of cayenne pepper

- ½ cup extra virgin olive oil
- 1 garlic clove, minced
- 2 handfuls mixed greens
- 1 avocado, pitted, peeled and cubed
- 1 red bell pepper, cut into thin strips
- 3 tablespoons melted coconut oil

Directions:

⇒ In a salad bowl, mix salad greens with avocado and pepper and leave aside for now.

⇒ In a bowl, mix lemon juice with mustard, garlic, mayo, pepper and a pinch of cayenne, stir well and leave aside.

⇒ Add olive oil gradually and whisk well again.

⇒ Rinse and pat dry scallops, put them in another bowl, add pepper to taste and 2 teaspoons cayenne and toss to coat.

⇒ Heat up a pan with the coconut oil over medium-high heat, add scallops, cook for 2 minutes on each side and transfer them to the bowl with the veggies.

⇒ Add mustard dressing you've made, toss to coat and serve.

Nutrition: calories 592, fat 46,3, carbs 23,8, fiber 28,9, protein 24,3

84) Pork and Lettuce Salad

Preparation Time: 10 minutes   **Cooking Time: 5 minutes**   **Servings:4**

Ingredients:

- 2 lettuce heads, torn
- 2 cups pork, already cooked and shredded
- 1 avocado, pitted, peeled and chopped
- 1 cup cherry tomatoes, cut in halves
- 1 green bell pepper, sliced
- 2 green onions, thinly sliced
- A pinch of sea salt

- Black pepper to taste
- Juice of ½ lime
- 1 tablespoon apple cider vinegar
- ¼ cup BBQ sauce
- 2 tablespoons extra virgin olive oil

Directions:

⇒ In a small bowl, mix oil with lime juice, vinegar, black pepper and BBQ sauce and whisk well.

⇒ Heat up a pan over medium heat, add pork meat and heat it up.

⇒ Meanwhile, in a salad bowl, mix lettuce leaves with tomatoes, bell pepper, avocado and green onions.

⇒ Add pork, drizzle the BBQ dressing, toss to coat and serve.

Nutrition: calories 349, fat 20,2, carbs 19,9, fiber 5,7, protein 24,3

85) Shrimp and Crab Salad

Preparation Time: 3 hours   **Cooking Time: 0 minutes**   **Servings:6**

Ingredients:

- 8 ounces, baby shrimp, already cooked, peeled, deveined and chopped
- 8 ounces crab meat, already cooked
- 2/3 cup homemade mayonnaise
- 2/3 cup yellow onion, chopped
- 2/3 cup celery, chopped

- 2 tablespoons Dijon mustard
- Black pepper to taste
- ¼ teaspoon onion powder
- ½ teaspoon garlic powder
- 1 tablespoon hot sauce

Directions:

⇒ In a salad bowl, mix shrimp with crab meat, onion, and celery.

⇒ In another bowl, mix mayo with mustard, pepper, onion powder, garlic powder and hot sauce and stir well.

⇒ Pour this over seafood salad, toss to coat and keep in the fridge for 3 hours before you serve it.

Nutrition: calories 198, fat 9,9, carbs 9, fiber 0,6, protein 16,8

86) Cilantro Beef Salad

Preparation Time: 10 minutes   **Cooking Time: 15 minutes**   **Servings:4**

Ingredients:

- 1 tablespoon chili powder
- 1 teaspoon onion powder
- ½ teaspoon garlic powder
- 1 teaspoon cumin, ground
- 2 teaspoons paprika
- 3 tablespoons olive oil
- A pinch of cayenne pepper
- 1 pound beef, ground
- 3 cups cilantro, chopped

- Juice from 1 lime
- A pinch of sea salt
- Black pepper to taste
- 1 romaine lettuce head, chopped
- 1 avocado, pitted, peeled and chopped
- 1 small red onion, chopped
- Some black olives, pitted and chopped
- 1 red bell pepper, chopped
- ½ cup Pico de gallo

Directions:

⇒ In a bowl, mix chili powder with paprika, onion and garlic powder, ½ teaspoon cumin, cayenne and some black pepper and stir.

⇒ Heat up a pan with 1 tablespoon oil over medium heat, add beef, stir and cook for 7 minutes.

⇒ Add spice mix, stir and cook until meat is done.

⇒ Meanwhile, in your food processor, blend 1 cup cilantro with lime juice, ½ teaspoon cumin, a pinch of salt, black pepper to taste and 2 tablespoons oil and pulse well.

⇒ In a salad bowl, mix lettuce leaves with avocado, 2 cups cilantro, onion, bell pepper, olives and Pico de gallo and stir.

⇒ Divide this between plates, top with beef and drizzle the salad dressing on top.

Nutrition: calories 464, fat 29,4, fiber 6,2, carbs 15,8, protein 27,1

87) Lemon Berries and Honeydew Salad

Preparation Time: 10 minutes   **Cooking Time: 0 minutes**   **Servings:6**

Ingredients:

- 1 cup blackberries, halved
- 2 cups honeydew, sliced
- 8 ounces prosciutto
- 3 tablespoons chives, chopped
- Juice of 1 lemon

- Zest from 1 lemon
- 1 shallot, chopped
- 2 cup cantaloupe, sliced
- A pinch of sea salt
- Black pepper to taste

Directions:

⇒ In a large salad bowl, mix blackberries with prosciutto, honeydew, cantaloupe, chives, lemon juice and zest, shallot, a pinch of sea salt and black pepper to taste, toss to coat and serve cold.

Nutrition: calories 107, fat 2,4, fiber 2,3, carbs 13,3, protein 9,1

88) Brussels Sprouts and Pecan Salad

Preparation Time: 10 minutes   **Cooking Time: 7 minutes**   **Servings:2**

Ingredients:

- 1 red onion, chopped
- 12 Brussels sprouts, sliced
- A pinch of sea salt
- Black pepper to taste
- 1 tablespoon olive oil

- 1/3 cup pecans, chopped
- ¼ cup raisins
- 2/3 cup hemp seeds
- ½ red apple, cored and chopped

Directions:

⇒ Heat up a pan with the oil over medium heat, add onion, stir and cook for a few minutes.

⇒ Add Brussels sprouts, cook for 4 minutes, take off heat and leave aside to cool down.

⇒ Add apple pieces, hemp seeds, raisins, a pinch of sea salt, black pepper and pecans, stir salad and serve.

Nutrition: calories 522, fat 34,8, fiber 10,2, carbs 42,1, protein 19,2

89) Lime Kale and Lettuce Salad

Preparation Time: 10 minutes   **Cooking Time: 0 minutes**   **Servings:1**

Ingredients:

- 1 carrot, grated
- A handful kale, chopped
- 1 small lettuce head, chopped
- 1 tablespoon tahini paste
- 1 tablespoon olive oil

- A pinch of sea salt
- Black pepper to taste
- Juice of ½ lime
- A pinch of garlic powder

Directions:

⇒ In a salad bowl, mix carrots with kale and lettuce leaves.

⇒ In a blender, mix tahini with a pinch of salt, black pepper, garlic powder, lime juice and oil and pulse well.

⇒ Pour this over salad, toss to coat well and serve.

Nutrition: calories 264, fat 22,2, fiber 3,8, carbs 16,9, protein 4,2

90) Chicken and Eggs Salad

Preparation Time: 10 minutes   **Cooking Time: 0 minutes**   **Servings:2**

Ingredients:

- 1 smoked chicken breast, sliced
- 2 handfuls lettuce leaves, torn
- 1 avocado, pitted, peeled and cubed

- 2 eggs, hard-boiled and halved
- A handful walnuts, chopped
- 2 tablespoons flaxseed oil

Directions:

⇒ In a salad bowl, mix lettuce with avocado, walnuts and chicken slices and toss.

⇒ Add eggs and oil, toss gently and serve.

Nutrition: calories 678, fat 49,7, fiber 10,7, carbs 20,9, protein 34,7

91) Balsamic Potato and Turkey Salad

Preparation Time: 10 minutes   **Cooking Time: 30 minutes**   **Servings:4**

Ingredients:

- 3 sweet potatoes, cubed
- 2 tablespoons coconut oil
- 4 garlic cloves, minced
- ½ pound turkey fillet, cut into thin slices
- Juice from 1 lime
- A pinch of sea salt
- Black pepper to taste

- 2 tablespoons balsamic vinegar
- 2 tablespoons olive oil
- A handful dill, chopped
- 2 green onions, chopped
- A pinch of cinnamon, ground
- A pinch of red pepper flakes

Directions:

⇒ Arrange turkey and sweet potatoes on a lined baking sheet, add garlic and coconut oil, toss well, place in the oven at 375 degrees F and bake for 30 minutes.

⇒ Meanwhile, in a bowl, mix vinegar with lime juice, olive oil, green onions, pepper flakes, dill, a pinch of sea salt, black pepper and cinnamon and stir well.

⇒ Transfer turkey and sweet potatoes to a salad bowl, add salad dressing, toss well and serve.

Nutrition: calories 316, fat 4,4, fiber 5,1, carbs 34,5, protein 13,4

92) Chicken and Olives Salad

Preparation Time: 10 minutes   **Cooking Time: 0 minutes**   **Servings:1**

Ingredients:

- 1 chicken breast, cooked and sliced
- 1 medium lettuce head, chopped
- 1 sweet potato, boiled and cubed
- 1 tablespoon pumpkin seeds

- 6 black olives, pitted and chopped
- 1 tablespoon olive oil
- 1 tablespoon balsamic vinegar

Directions:

⇒ In a salad bowl, mix chicken breast slices with lettuce, sweet potato, pumpkin seeds, olives, olive oil and balsamic vinegar, stir well and serve right away.

⇒

Nutrition: calories 760, fat 30,4, fiber 8,4, carbs 43,1, protein 78,3

93) Salmon and Cucumber Salad

Preparation Time: 10 minutes   **Cooking Time: 5 minutes**   **Servings:2**

Ingredients:

- 1 lettuce head, chopped
- 2 salmon fillets
- 1 tablespoon olive oil
- 1 tablespoon coconut aminos

- 1 avocado, pitted, peeled and sliced
- 1 cucumber, sliced
- A pinch of sea salt
- Black pepper to taste

Directions:

⇒ Heat up a pan with the oil over medium-high heat, add salmon fillets skin side down, cook for 3 minutes, flip and cook for 2 minutes more.

⇒ In a salad bowl, mix lettuce with cucumber, avocado, a pinch of salt, black pepper and coconut aminos and stir.

⇒ Flake salmon using a fork, add to salad, drizzle some of the oil from the pan, toss to coat and serve.

Nutrition: calories 550, fat 38,1, fiber 8,5, carbs 20, protein 38,2

94) Lettuce, Kale and Radish Salad

Preparation Time: 10 minutes   **Cooking Time: 0 minutes**   **Servings:3**

Ingredients:

- 1 lettuce head, chopped
- A handful kale, chopped
- A handful steamed broccoli
- A handful walnuts, chopped
- 8 cherry tomatoes, halved
- A handful radishes, chopped
- 1 tablespoon lemon juice
- 8 dates, chopped
- A drizzle of olive oil

Directions:

⇒ In a salad bowl, mix lettuce with kale, broccoli, walnuts, tomatoes, radishes and dates.

⇒ In smaller bowl, mix lemon juice with olive oil and whisk well.

⇒ Add this to salad, toss to coat and serve.

Nutrition: calories 771, fat 35,2, fiber 36,2, carbs 112,4, protein 21,4

95) Tomato and Mayo Salad

Preparation Time: 10 minutes   **Cooking Time: 0 minutes**   **Servings:4**

Ingredients:

- 1 bunch kale, chopped
- 12 cherry tomatoes, halved
- 2 handfuls microgreens
- 3 tablespoons Paleo mayonnaise
- 1 teaspoon mustard

Directions:

⇒ In a salad bowl, mix tomatoes with greens and kale.

⇒ In a small bowl, mix mayo with mustard and whisk well.

⇒ Add this to salad, toss to coat and serve.

Nutrition: calories 145, fat 8,5, fiber 4,9, carbs 16, protein 4

Chapter 9 -   Dessert Recipes

96) Maple Rhubarb Bowls

Preparation Time: 10 minutes   **Cooking Time: 5 minutes**   **Servings:3**

Ingredients:

- Juice of 1 lemon
- Some thin lemon zest strips
- 1 and ½ cup maple syrup

- 4 and ½ cups rhubarbs cut into medium pieces.
- 1 vanilla bean
- 1 and ½ cups water

Directions:

⇒ Put the water in a saucepan.

⇒ Add maple syrup, vanilla bean, lemon juice and lemon zest.

⇒ Stir, bring to a boil and add rhubarb.

⇒ Reduce heat, simmer for 5 minutes, take off heat and transfer rhubarb to a bowl.

⇒ Allow liquid to cool down, discard vanilla bean and serve.

Nutrition: calories 297, fat 0,6, fiber 2,8, carbs 75,3, protein 1,4

97) Maple Cobbler

Preparation Time: 10 minutes   **Cooking Time: 30 minutes**   **Servings:5**

Ingredients:

- ¾ cup maple syrup
- 6 cups strawberries, halved
- 1 tablespoon lemon juice
- ½ cup coconut flour

- 1/4 teaspoon baking soda
- ½ cup water
- 3 and ½ tablespoons coconut oil
- A drizzle of avocado oil

Directions:

⇒ Grease a baking dish with a drizzle of avocado oil and leave aside.

⇒ In a bowl, mix strawberries with maple syrup, sprinkle some flour and add lemon juice.

⇒ Stir very well and pour into baking dish.

⇒ In another bowl, mix flour with baking soda and stir well.

⇒ Add coconut and mix until the whole thing crumbles in your hands.

⇒ Add ½ cup water and spread over strawberries.

⇒ Place in the oven at 375 degrees F and bake for 30 minutes.

⇒ Take cobbler out of the oven, leave aside for 10 minutes and then serve.

Nutrition: calories 318, fat 11,2, fiber 9,5, carbs 55, protein 3,2

98) Cocoa Almond Bowls

Preparation Time: 3 hours   **Cooking Time:**   **Servings:4**

Ingredients:

- 1 cup almond milk
- 2 avocados, peeled and pitted
- ¾ cup cocoa powder
- 1 teaspoon vanilla extract

- ¾ cup maple syrup
- ¼ teaspoon cinnamon
- Walnuts chopped for serving

Directions:

⇒ Put avocados in a kitchen blender and pulse well.

⇒ Add cocoa powder, almond milk, maple syrup, cinnamon and vanilla extract and pulse well again.

⇒ Pour into serving bowls, top with walnuts and keep in the fridge for 2-3 hours before you serve it.

Nutrition: calories 536, fat 36,1, fiber 12,9, carbs 60,7, protein 6,2

99) Dates and Plums Smoothie Bowls

Preparation Time: 2 hours   **Cooking Time: 0 minutes**   **Servings:4**

Ingredients:

- 1 cup dates, pitted and chopped
- 3 cups plums, chopped
- 2 and ½ cups water
- 1 teaspoon lemon juice

Directions:

⇒ Put dates and plums in a food processor and blend well.

⇒ Add water gradually and pulse a few more times.

⇒ Add lemon juice, pulse for a few more seconds, transfer to a bowl and keep in the freezer for 2 hours.

⇒ Scoop into dessert cups and serve right away!

Nutrition: calories 148, fat 0,3, carbs 39,4, fiber 4,3, protein 1,5

100)   Green Avocado Bowls

Preparation Time: 6 minutes   **Cooking Time:**   **Servings:4**

Ingredients:

- ½ cup coconut water
- 1 and ½ cup avocado, chopped
- 2 tablespoons green tea powder
- 2 teaspoons lime zest
- 1 tablespoon honey
- Melted coconut butter for serving
- 1 mango thinly sliced for serving

Directions:

⇒ In a blender, mix water with avocado, green tea powder and lime zest and pulse well.

⇒ Add honey and pulse again well.

⇒ Transfer to a bowl, top with coconut butter spread all over and serve with sliced mango.

Nutrition: calories 216, fat 15,7, fiber 8,6, carbs 18,4, protein 4,7

101)   Maple Ice Cream

Preparation Time: 2 hours   **Cooking Time: 3 minutes**   **Servings:8**

Ingredients:

- 1 tablespoon arrowroot powder
- 2 cans coconut milk
- ¼ teaspoon vanilla beans
- 1 tablespoon water
- 1/3 cup pure maple syrup
- 1/3 cup coconut nectar

Directions:

⇒ Fill 1/3 of a bowl with ice cubes, place another bowl on top and leave aside for now.

⇒ Pour coconut milk in a saucepan, reserve 2 tablespoons, put them in a bowl, mix with arrowroot starch and stir well.

⇒ Add arrowroot mix of coconut milk to the saucepan and stir.

⇒ Also add vanilla beans, maple syrup and coconut nectar, stir well, place on stove and heat up over medium heat.

⇒ Stir well, bring to a boil, boil for 2 minutes, take off heat and pour into the bowl you've placed over the ice.

⇒ Add water, stir well and leave aside for 1 hour and 30 minutes.

⇒ Pour this into your ice cream machine and turn on.

⇒ Pour into a container, place in the freezer and leave it there for 20 minutes.

⇒ Serve right away!

Nutrition: calories 151, fat 14,5, fiber 1,5, carbs 6, protein 1,4

102) Fruity Cashew Cream

Preparation Time: 6 hours and 10 minutes   **Cooking Time: 0 minutes**   **Servings:6**

Ingredients:

- 1 cup apples, chopped
- 1 cup pineapple, chopped
- 1 cup chickoo, chopped
- 1 cup melon, chopped
- 1 cup papaya, chopped
- ½ teaspoon vanilla powder
- ¾ cup cashews
- Stevia to the taste
- Some cold water

Directions:

⇒ Put cashews in a bowl, add some water on top, leave aside for 6 hours, drain them and put them in a food processor.

⇒ Blend them well and add cold water to cover them.

⇒ Also add stevia and vanilla, blend some more and keep in the fridge for now.

⇒ In a bowl, arrange a layer of mixed apples with pineapples, melon, papaya and chickoo

⇒ Add a layer of cold cashew paste, another layer of fruits, another one of cashew paste and to with a layer of fruits.

⇒ Serve right away!

Nutrition: calories 282, fat 1867, fiber 3,1, carbs 26,5, protein 6,7

103) Chia and Almond Pudding

Preparation Time: 2 hours   **Cooking Time: 0 minutes**   **Servings:4**

Ingredients:

- 2 tablespoons cocoa powder
- 1 cup almond milk
- 1 tablespoon chia seeds
- A pinch of salt
- ½ teaspoon vanilla extract

Directions:

⇒ In a bowl, mix cocoa powder, almond milk, vanilla extract and chia seeds and stir well until they blend.

⇒ Transfer to a dessert glass, place in the fridge for 2 hours and then serve.

Nutrition: calories 180, fat 16,8, fiber 4,7, carbs 7,9, protein 3

104) Matcha Muffins

Preparation Time: 40 minutes   **Cooking Time: 0 minutes**   **Servings:4**

Ingredients:

- 5 tablespoons almond flour
- ½ cup soft coconut butter
- ¾ cup cocoa powder
- ¼ cup cocoa butter
- 1 teaspoon matcha powder (and some more for the topping)
- 3 tablespoons maple syrup
- 1 teaspoon coconut oil
- Cocoa nibs

Directions:

⇒ In a bowl, mix coconut butter with almond flour, maple syrup and matcha powder, stir, cover and keep in the fridge for 10 minutes.

⇒ Put cocoa butter and cocoa powder in a bowl and mix with coconut oil.

⇒ Spoon 2 teaspoons of this melted mix in a muffin liner.

⇒ Repeat this with 7 other muffin liners.

⇒ Take 1 tablespoon matcha mix and shape a ball, place in a muffin liner, press to flatten it and repeat this with the rest of the muffin liners.

⇒ Top each with 1 tablespoon cocoa mass and spread evenly.

⇒ Sprinkle some matcha powder all over muffins.

⇒ Add cocoa nibs on top of each, place them in the freezer and keep there until they are solid.

⇒ Take them out of the freezer, leave at room temperature for a few minutes and serve.

Nutrition: calories 522, fat 46,5, fiber 13,3, carbs 32,4, protein 7,7

105) Almond Ice Cream

Preparation Time: 10 minutes   **Cooking Time: 6 minutes**   **Servings:6**

Ingredients:

For the caramel sauce:

- ¾ cup stevia
- ½ cup coconut milk
- 2 tablespoons maple syrup
- 1 teaspoon vanilla extract

For the ice cream:

- 12 ounces firm almond cheese
- 1 can coconut milk
- 100 drops liquid stevia
- 2 teaspoons guar

Directions:

⇒ In a pan, heat over medium-high heat ½ cup coconut milk, ¾ cup stevia and maple syrup.

⇒ Stir well, bring to a boil, reduce heat to low and simmer for 3-4 minutes.

⇒ Take off heat, add vanilla extract, stir and leave in the fridge to cool down completely.

⇒ In a food processor, mix coconut milk, almond cheese, a pinch of salt and the caramel and pulse well.

⇒ Add guar and blend again well.

⇒ Take mix from the fridge and transfer to an ice cream maker.

⇒ When the ice cream is done, transfer to bowls and serve with caramel on top.

Nutrition: calories 250, fat 17,6, fiber 0,9, carbs 23,7, protein 7,8

106) Pumpkin Pudding

Preparation Time: 1 hour and 20 minutes   **Cooking Time: 0 minutes**   **Servings:4**

Ingredients:

- 1 cup almond milk
- ½ cup pumpkin puree
- 2 tablespoons maple syrup
- ½ cup coconut milk
- ½ teaspoon cinnamon powder
- ½ teaspoon vanilla extract
- ¼ teaspoon ginger, grated
- ¼ cup chia seeds

Directions:

⇒ In a bowl, mix almond milk with coconut milk, pumpkin puree, cinnamon, maple syrup, vanilla and ginger and stir well.

⇒ Add chia seeds, stir and leave aside for 20 minutes.

⇒ Divide into 4 glasses, cover and keep in the fridge for 1 hour.

Nutrition: calories 314, fat 25,9, fiber 7,8, carbs 20,3, protein 4,8

107) Cashew Fudge

Preparation Time: 30 minutes   **Cooking Time: 0 minutes**   **Servings:4**

Ingredients:

- 1/3 cup natural cashew butter
- 1 and ½ tablespoons coconut oil
- 2 tablespoons coconut butter
- 5 tablespoons lemon juice
- ½ teaspoon lemon zest
- A pinch of salt
- 1 tablespoons maple syrup

Directions:

⇒ In a bowl, mix cashew butter with coconut one, coconut oil, lemon juice, lemon zest, a pinch of salt and maple syrup and stir until you obtain a creamy mix.

⇒ Line a muffin tray with some parchment paper, scoop 1 tablespoon of fudge mix in each of the 10 pieces, place in the freezer and keep the for a few hours.

⇒ Take out of the fridge 20 minutes before you serve them.

Nutrition: calories 161, fat 14, fiber 2,9, carbs 11,2, protein 3,7

108) Hemp and Berry Bars

Preparation Time: 30 minutes   **Cooking Time: 0 minutes**   **Servings:6**

Ingredients:

- ¼ cup cocoa nibs
- 1 cup almonds, soaked for at least 3 hours
- 2 tablespoons cocoa powder
- ¼ cup hemp seeds

- ¼ cup goji berries
- ¼ cup coconut, shredded
- 8 dates, pitted and soaked

Directions:

⇒ Put almonds in a food processor and blend them well.

⇒ Add hemp seeds, cocoa nibs, cocoa powder, goji, coconut and blend well.

⇒ Add dates gradually and blend some more.

⇒ Transfer mix to a parchment paper, spread and press it.

⇒ Cut in equal pieces and serve after you've kept them in the fridge for 30 minutes.

Nutrition: calories 304, fat 16,8, fiber 6,1, carbs 32,8, protein 8,4

Chapter 10 -   Paleo Gillian's Meal Plan – for Men

Day 1

2) Coconut Berry Smoothie | Calories 222

16) Herbed Chicken and Olives Stew | Calories 553

32) Garlic Potato and Pine Nuts Cream | Calories 445

43) Banana and Walnut Snack | Calories 464

51) Baked Kale Bowls | Calories 9

64) Coffee Steaks | Calories 621

Total Calories 2314

Day 3

7) Coconut Smoothie | Calories 336

23) Chicken, Tomato and Kale Soup | Calories 1227

33) Asparagus and Green Onions Mix | Calories 141

50) Chicken Platter | Calories 485

55) Salsa Pork Mix | Calories 1013

75) Clams and Apple Mix | Calories 610

Total Calories 3812

Day 5

13) Poached Eggs with Artichokes and Lemon Sauce | Calories 1130

19) Nutmeg Coconut and Squash Cream | Calories 245

38) Balsamic Peppers and Capers Mix | Calories 123

45) Thyme Zucchini Fries | Calories 106

58) Balsamic Pork Mix | Calories 271

83) Cayenne Scallops and Avocado Salad | Calories 592

Total Calories 2467

Day 7

8) Walnut and Hemp Bowls | Calories 403

25) Mustard Mushroom Cream | Calories 171

41) Paprika Okra Mix | Calories 107

49) Dehydrated Beef Bites | Calories 273

61) Turkey with Peppers and Tomatoes | Calories 306

87) Lemon Berries and Honeydew Salad | Calories 107

Total Calories 1367

Day 2

3) Lemon Kale Smoothie | Calories 138

19) Nutmeg Coconut and Squash Cream | Calories 245

35) Garlic and Basil Tomatoes | Calories 91

42) Hot Artichoke Bowls | Calories 109

63) Steaks and Pico de Gallo | Calories 285

77) Shrimp and Parsley Mix | Calories 374

Total Calories 1242

Day 4

10) Coconut Orange Bowls | Calories 672

30) Shallot and Cauliflower Cream | Calories 291

40) Lemon Chili Cabbage | Calories 118

48) Coconut Chicken Bites | Calories 330

60) Garlic Pork and Strawberries | Calories 981

90) Chicken and Eggs Salad | Calories 678

Total Calories 3070

Day 6

5) Mint Berry Smoothie | Calories 59

28) Coconut Zucchini Cream | Calories 122

36) Garlic Spinach | Calories 146

47) Turkey Balls | Calories 71

56) Smoked Pork Ribs | Calories 1483

69) Shrimp and Radish Cakes | Calories 406

Total Calories 2287

Chapter 11 -   Conclusion

Always remember to consult with your medical professional before starting any dietary path.

I hope this book can be the springboard to start your long term transformation journey

You can check out (or give away) the other books in the series, just search for Kaylee Gillian.

Regards

Kaylee

CPSIA information can be obtained
at www.ICGtesting.com
Printed in the USA
LVHW020806160621
690358LV00012B/1927